Infection Control

A PSYCHOSOCIAL APPROACH TO CHANGING PRACTICE

For Una and John

Infection Control

A PSYCHOSOCIAL APPROACH TO CHANGING PRACTICE

Edited by

PAUL ELLIOTT

MA, BSc, PGCEA, RGN, EN(M), ISM Cert, FRIPH, FHEA
Senior Lecturer in Adult Nursing and Infection Prevention
Department of Nursing and Applied Clinical Studies
Canterbury Christ Church University
Canterbury

Forewords by

SHEILA MORGAN
Nurse Consultant in Infection Prevention and Control

PROFESSOR MARK WILCOX
Professor of Medical Microbiology
University of Leeds

and

DR ROBERT C SPENCER
Consultant Medical Microbiologist
Past Chairman of the Hospital Infection Society (2001–2007)

Radcliffe Publishing
Oxford • New York

Radcliffe Publishing Ltd
18 Marcham Road
Abingdon
Oxon OX14 1AA
United Kingdom

www.radcliffe-oxford.com
Electronic catalogue and worldwide online ordering facility.

British Library Cataloguing in Publication Data

A catalogue record for this book is available from the British Library.

ISBN-13: 978 185775 612 8

Typeset by Pindar New Zealand, Auckland, New Zealand
Printed and bound by Cadmus Communications, USA

Contents

Foreword

In the last decade the re-emphasis for sound infection prevention and control knowledge and practices, which are essential for public health, to be restored at the cornerstone of clinical management have been at the forefront of government policy. With the requirement to reduce and minimise the incidence of healthcare associated infection (HCAI), the ever-changing pattern of infection, in conjunction with the emergence of multiple antibiotic resistant micro-organisms, have emphasised the need for all healthcare workers to understand and consistently apply sound principles to their clinical practice to provide a high-quality and safe patient focused service.

This book addresses the complex issue of why an individual may not comply with policy and practices. It encourages the reader to reflect and explore their personal attitudes, and that of others, in the application of infection and control practice, suggesting why certain approaches do not work and providing insights into what motivates an individual to do well and how these factors can be encapsulated into successful models for bringing about changes in attitudes and practice.

This publication provides an informative, thought provoking reference for undergraduate and graduate study in addition to all healthcare professionals employed across the whole health economy.

Sheila Morgan
Nurse Consultant in Infection Prevention and Control
January 2009

Foreword

Infection prevention is everyone's 'business' in the healthcare setting. The raised profile of infection has most recently been underpinned by changes in UK law that require healthcare institutions to make infection prevention mandatory rather than an optional extra. Increasing emphasis on safety and high quality of healthcare will quite rightly make healthcare-associated infection even less acceptable.

To anyone involved in infection prevention and control, whether at an operational or strategic level, the failure of healthcare workers, patients and visitors to adhere to what at face level appear to be straightforward infection prevention recommendations remains both a conundrum and impediment to minimising the risk of infection transmission. Despite the common sense mantra that underlies much infection-control practice, considerable time and effort are expended at achieving compliance, notably with hand hygiene recommendations. The hardness of the nut that is achieving universal compliance by healthcare workers with infection prevention and control procedures shows that reliance on practical measures and exhortations alone to crack this problem is insufficient.

Paul Elliott has drawn together a thought provoking (pardon the pun) collection of topics that together explain the psychology of infection prevention and control. This is not simply a book about psychology; it is about how to change and improve practice written by people who understand the trade of infection prevention and control. Reflection exercises are cleverly used throughout the text to provoke the reader to think of their own experiences in and their practice of healthcare. The reader is led into considering how improvements can be made to the delivery of infection prevention and control, and at the same time to understand why the way we think ultimately determines the likelihood of their success. The reader is helped through each reflection exercise by the use of clear and concise explanations in a non-confrontational way. The effect is to make the reader analyse and critique him/herself and the way we do things now.

This approach aims to help us understand the ways in which infection-control practice and service delivery by an organisation can be optimised, and most importantly improvements sustained. It is surprising when the psychology of infection control is considered for more than a fleeting moment (as has been the tendency in the past) why it has taken so long for the penny to drop. Optimising infection prevention and control in an organisation can only be achieved by optimising the behaviours of the staff (and patients and visitors), who are the organisation.

I congratulate Paul Elliott (as he puts it) for challenging the status quo with respect to the way we think about infection prevention and control. Recognising the problem of infection risk, designing ways of preventing microbe transmission and measuring success are not enough to optimise infection prevention and control practice. We need to think better. This book challenges and helps healthcare professionals to do that.

Professor Mark Wilcox
Professor of Medical Microbiology, University of Leeds
Consultant, Head of Microbiology and Clinical Director of Pathology,
Leeds Teaching Hospitals, Leeds, UK
Lead on *Clostridium difficile* infection for the Regional Microbiology
Network of the Health Protection Agency in England
January 2009

Foreword

The problems posed by healthcare associated infections (HCAIs) have, in recent years, achieved an unprecedented impact in the eyes of not only healthcare workers of all professions, but also the general public and political parties of all persuasions.

This is not a situation unique to the United Kingdom, but an international one with the World Health Organization leading the way via their World Alliance for Patient Safety. Suggested ways to combat and solve the problems of HCAIs are myriad with an amazing range of possible solutions from 'bare below the elbows', ridding doctors of ties, 'a man thing', antibiotic policies, antimicrobial paints and surface coatings to name but a few. Some have potential value and are evidence based, whilst others will fall by the wayside. Everyone I know who is professionally involved with HCAIs, whether due to methicillin-resistant *Staphylococcus aureus* (MRSA) or *Clostridium difficile*, are united in identifying the principle villain – the lack of adequate and effective hand washing. In 1847 Ignaz Semmelweis, a Hungarian physician, discovered that by the simple expedient of hand washing in obstetric practice, the incidence of puerperal or childbed fever could be drastically reduced. Despite achieving dramatic reductions in the incidence of this fatal sepsis at the maternity clinic of the Vienna General Hospital, his hypothesis was ignored, rejected and ridiculed. One hundred and sixty years later, despite the fact that hand washing is recognised as the key to any successful infection control initiative, there still remains an amazing reluctance from healthcare workers, especially doctors, to comply with this simple, basic remedy. Why? Belatedly the role of behavioural influences on the practice of infection control, as to whether it is successful or not, is being increasingly recognised as a key facet, on both sides of the Atlantic. It is therefore timely and most welcome that a book devoted to the psychosocial approach to achieving a change in practice has surfaced. The author asks the reader to question their own behaviour and how it impacts on the behaviour of others. A cry goes out for opinion leaders and role models, be they Senior Nurses or Doctors. At the same time the patient, or in the modern euphemism, the consumer, also needs to be aware of these psychosocial approaches. As with the current NHS Wash Your Hands campaign it is indeed safe for the patient to ask. If we as healthcare professionals wish to maintain our cherished patient–doctor/nurse relationship, then a perusal through this book will help preserve it for some time to come.

Dr Robert C Spencer
Consultant Medical Microbiologist
Past Chairman of the Hospital Infection Society (2001–2007)
January 2009

Preface

There can be no doubt that the infection-control behaviour of health and social care workers, irrespective of their profession, role or appointment, has a significant impact upon patients and clients. Over many years much has been published or discussed at conferences worldwide regarding the nature and cause of non-adherence to the likes of standard precautions. However, for the most part, what has been stated is simply repetitive in identifying that a problem of non-adherence exists and where potential solutions are offered they are, for the most part, biomedical in nature. With a few exceptions there has been a complete failure to recognise and identify the psychological and social issues involved within the context of a biopsychosocial approach.

In order to enhance your reading of this book, each of the chapters has a number of reflection exercises. These exercises have been designed to challenge your assumptions and beliefs about infection control and your own infection-control practice. You may find that in undertaking these exercises you recognise things about yourself and your infection-control practice that you do not like and it may make you feel uncomfortable. Your human reaction may be to put the book down or not to undertake the reflection exercises. However, I hope that you will not do this. Part of gaining the maximum benefit from this book is for you to become more aware of your own and others' infection-control practice.

As you read through the book you will see that the same references, diagrams, lists and explanation boxes appear within a number of chapters. There are four reasons for this:

1 These are related to sources, theories and approaches, which are central to the psychosocial nature of poor infection control practice.
2 I have attempted to minimise the number of sources, theories and approaches used within the book so that you should not be overwhelmed by excessive amounts of material.
3 The main themes that underpin this book are about how people think and the concepts that underpin such thinking – both of which are highly

complex. Therefore my intention has been to enhance your understanding rather than confuse you.

4 Repeating the various lists and explanation boxes, etc., in the relevant chapters is to prevent your reading of the book being disrupted by having to refer back to previous chapters to find a particular source, theory or approach.

Finally, in writing this book, along with contributions from a number of health and social care professionals – all of whom are colleagues and have considerable expertise in their fields – I have deliberately set out to challenge the status quo and to push the frontiers of your thinking in relation to infection control. In doing this, it is my hope that you will find what you read to be challenging and interesting. I have also attempted to provide a text that closes a gap where infection-control research, education and practice leaves much to be desired.

LEARNING OUTCOMES

In reading this book you will have the opportunity to:
1 reflect upon a range psychosocial theories and approaches that impact upon the infection-control behaviour of health and social care workers;
2 reflect upon your own infection control behaviour and why, on occasions, you fail to adopt standard precautions from a psychosocial perspective;
3 reflect upon the clinical, legal and human rights issues related to your own and others' infection-control practice;
4 reflect upon the issues that surround changing infection-control behaviour;
5 reflect upon a number of strategies that can serve to enhance consistent safe infection-control practice;
6 reflect upon the importance of challenging the status quo in facilitating safe infection-control practice;
7 reflect upon the public's right to know the risks they are at from poor infection-control practice by you and others;
8 enhance your awareness of the fact that the way you and others think about infection control will directly influence the quality of your practice and the degree to which you inflict harm upon patients, clients and colleagues.

Paul Elliott
January 2009

About the editor

Paul Elliott's initial nurse education and the first half of his professional career was spent in the Royal Air Force undertaking a variety of roles culminating in an aero-medical evacuation/emergency practitioner role within operational unit medical centres and squadrons of tactical support helicopters during field deployments. After leaving the RAF in 1985, he held appointments within accident and emergency and medical admissions settings in the National Health Service in the UK. In 1991, he moved into full-time healthcare education where his career has developed initially with the Buckinghamshire College of Nursing and Midwifery, then the University of Surrey, and currently with Canterbury Christ Church University. His primary research interests are in the psychosocial aspects of infection prevention/control, and he has had several publications in that area.

List of contributors

Sue Clark MSc (Public Health), BSc (Hons), PG Cert (L&T), IC Cert, RGN
Senior Lecturer
Department of Nursing and Applied Clinical Studies
Canterbury Christ Church University
Medway Campus, UK

Lynn Parker MSc Nursing Studies, PGCE for Nurses, RN
Co-founder Healthcare A2Z and Clinical Advisor
Comberton, Cambridgeshire, UK

Bernie Warren PhD
Professor, Drama in Education and Community
School of Dramatic Art
University of Windsor
Windsor, Ontario, Canada

Ben Waters BA, PGDipL
Solicitor and Senior Lecturer in Law
Department of Law and Criminal Justice Studies
Faculty of Social and Applied Sciences
Canterbury Christ Church University, UK

Janet Wiseman PhD, MSc (Mental Health), Dip Social Work
Senior Lecturer in Social Work
Department of Social Work, Community and Mental Health
Faculty of Health and Social Care
Canterbury Christ Church University, UK

Acknowledgements

I would like to acknowledge and offer my thanks to the following:

To each of the contributors for their chapters and their understanding regarding the length of time it has taken to complete this book: Bernie Warren, Lynn Parker, Ben Waters, Sue Clark, Janet Wiseman.

To my wife, Annie, for being a sounding block; for her thoughts regarding the content of this book and for helping to keep me on track.

To Gill Nineham at Radcliffe Publishing for her support and understanding with regards to my completing the book.

To Carrie Sanders as my Head of Department for her support in terms of time to complete the book.

To Natasha Lewis for giving up her own time to help me format the structure of the book.

Without the support that each of the above individuals gave me in their own ways, I very much doubt this book would have come to fruition. Thank you one and all.

SECTION 1

Outlining the major issues

INTRODUCTION

In this section we introduce three perspectives:

1   The psychosocial nature of infection control (Chapters 1, 4, 5 and 6) with a specific emphasis on standard precautions. Within this context, Chapter 1 is intended to provide you with a general introduction to the subject matter. Chapter 4 introduces biomedical and biopsychosocial models and links them to infection control. Chapter 5 introduces a range of individual psychosocial theories and approaches that impact upon all health and social care professionals and influence their infection control behaviour. Chapter 6 revisits the theories and approaches presented within Chapter 5, and aims to show how none of these theories and approaches exist in isolation, but all act together to influence infection control behaviour.

2   Chapter 2 offers a perspective from the clinical setting and reflects the complexity of clinical infection control practice. This chapter also aims to provide you with an understanding of the complex issues infection control specialists are presented with on a daily basis.

3   Chapter 3 aims to introduce you to the legal issues related to infection control and the consequences of failing to practice in a safe and professional manner. For the most part, many workers in health and social areas are exceptionally complacent with regard to the legal consequences of their infection control behaviour.

CHAPTER 1

The psychosocial nature of infection control

In this chapter, my intention is to introduce the psychosocial nature of infection control and highlight some of the issues as I see them. To start at the beginning, what is actually meant by 'psychosocial issues'? In essence, these are the psychological and social issues that impact upon an individual's ability to undertake safe infection control practice. To date, strategies aimed at reducing healthcare-acquired infection and improving the infection control practices of health and social care professionals have centred on the physical. For example, *the unilateral implementation of prescriptive rules by management in the form of policies and procedures, who have the misguided belief that these will promote appropriate behaviour.*

REFLECTION EXERCISE 1.1

Think about the example above and consider why it would be unlikely to promote consistent and safe infection control behaviour.

In undertaking this exercise think about how you would feel having something imposed upon you over which you were not consulted.

Although such strategies may be worthwhile in themselves, they are physically orientated and unless they are linked to the psychological and social issues involved they will fail to facilitate safe infection control behaviour in the long term. Further, physically orientated strategies in isolation will not make any long-term difference to the way individuals think about infection control; for example, within the context of the adoption of standard precautions (*see* List 1.1).

LIST 1.1 STANDARD PRECAUTIONS

There are a number of standard precautions involved in infection control:

1   **Recognising the need** to adopt standard precautions is the most important aspect. Failing to recognise the need is governed by the way an individual thinks, which will, in turn, impact upon their perception of the relevance and importance of such precautions. If an individual perceives standard precautions as being irrelevant, unimportant or of a lesser priority, then the potential for non-adherence is significantly increased.

2   **Hand hygiene** is vital in facilitating the prevention and reduction of healthcare-acquired infections. Hand hygiene must be carried out frequently by individuals who are constantly reflecting upon the principle of what they have just done and what they are about to do now. If the *just done* constitutes a risk to themselves or others then appropriate hand hygiene must be undertaken prior to proceeding to the *do now*. Also, consideration must be given to the full hand hygiene process (*see* List 1.3).

3   **Hand cleansing rubs/gels** are an effective method of hand decontamination in the short term. However, they should never be perceived as an absolute substitute for the adoption of formal hand hygiene using the hand hygiene process.

4   **Disposable aprons** can provide some protection for the wearer. However, they should never be perceived as an absolute barrier and must be changed frequently. As a general rule the *just done, do now* approach should be adopted at all times.

5   **Disposable gloves** must always be worn when handling body fluids or any contaminated substance/materials. As a general rule, if in doubt wear gloves. Management and/or colleagues should not presume to ridicule or restrict an individual's decision to wear gloves.

6   **Skin trauma** must be dealt with in accordance with the employer's policies and procedures, and in accordance with health and safety laws. All trauma to the skin, irrespective of how minor, must be cleaned, dried, covered and reported. It is a legal requirement that an accident/incident form is completed and individuals should report to either the Occupational Health Department or to Accident and Emergency.

7   **The eyes** should be protected where there is either a potential or actual risk of

flying debris or splashes of body fluids/harmful substances. Individuals must determine for themselves when the wearing of appropriate eye protection is necessary. Management should not presume to restrict such determinations or they may be in contravention of an individual's human rights under Articles 1 and 10 (Wilkinson and Caulfield 2001)(*see* List 1.4).

8 **Sharps** are dangerous and will cause harm. A sharp may be defined as anything that can either penetrate or cause trauma to the skin. An injury from a sharp may have consequences for the remainder of an individual's life. Always handle sharps with caution for your own safety and that of those around you. The rule is that if you have been using sharps then you are responsible to clear up what you have used and dispose of the sharps correctly. If you fail to do this you are acting in an unprofessional and unethical manner.

9 **Spillages** of any kind can be hazardous to the health and wellbeing of you and others. The rule is, if you cause the spillage then you clean it up or ensure it is dealt with in the correct way. Your employer's policies and procedures for dealing with spillages must be adhered to at all times.

10 **Waste materials** can be divided into three categories: household, clinical and contaminated/hazardous. However, all categories of waste should be handled with caution as each one is capable of increasing the risk of cross infection and causing harm to yourself and others. Your employer's policies and procedures for the disposal of waste must be adhered to at all times.

11 **Linen**, like waste materials, must be handled with care due to the increased potential for cross infection. When handling soiled or contaminated linen appropriate protective clothing should be worn. With regard to the handling of clean linen, the *just done, do now* approach should be adopted. Your employer's policies and procedures for the handling of linen must be adhered to at all times.

12 **Food handling** is an activity that we all do either at a personal level for our own consumption or at a social level for consumption by others. The mishandling of food is a prime source of cross infection and the use of appropriate protective clothing and meticulous hand hygiene is essential using the *just done, do now* approach.

13 **Environmental contamination**, although not always visible to the human eye, is always present. Therefore regular and rigorous cleaning of healthcare environments is essential to reduce the risk of cross infection. Although many people involved in the provision of healthcare perceive such environmental cleaning as being the role of designated cleaners, such a role is arguably the responsibility of everyone. The rule is that if you cause the contamination, you clean it up or ensure it is cleaned up in an appropriate manner. It is

both unethical and unprofessional to simply leave contamination with the expectation that it is someone else's responsibility to clean it up.

14 **Personal hygiene** of those involved in the provision of healthcare and recipients of healthcare is an essential measure where the reduction of cross infection is concerned.

If a strategy fails to impact upon an individual's thinking, then the potential for that strategy to fail will be high, which has been identified by Reason, Parker and Lawton (1998) and Lawton and Parker (1999). Therefore, simply presenting an individual with the written word as decreed by others will not change their thinking. For example, take a policy that tells you to undertake standard precautions. Although health and social care professionals may understand the importance of this policy, the reasons for their non-adherence may be the result of how well the policy is designed, presented, written (in terms of the language used) and implemented. Consideration must be given to each of these factors with regard to:

➤ the physical appearance of the policy (is it eye catching?);
➤ the psychological impact of the policy upon an individual (does the individual feel it has importance for them?);
➤ the social impression the policy gives (does the policy have relevance to the individual's area of practice?);
➤ the individual's sense of ownership (were they consulted as a part of the development process?).

Prescriptive rules, such as policies or procedures, are generally presented as orders and instructions as opposed to information intended to facilitate personal safety. However, human nature being what it is means that we dislike being ordered or instructed, so we usually react negatively rather than respond positively to prescriptive rules. In addition, as Reason, Parker and Lawton (1998) and Lawton and Parker (1999) further indicate, the greater the number of prescriptive rules that are imposed upon us the greater the degree of our non-adherence. Further, if the prescriptive rule we are presented with conflicts with our past experience, it may also lead to non-adherence. This can occur, for example, when the policy conflicts with what our parents or peer group believes about hand hygiene.

Failing to recognise the psychosocial issues involved in infection control is not restricted to any particular profession, organisation or society – it is a global problem that impacts upon us all. Subsequently, infection control is everyone's responsibility, despite the fact that many health and social care professionals regularly ignore that responsibility. For example:

➤ **In the case of a clinical practitioner:** 'I am too busy caring for my patients to worry about undertaking standard precautions or doing what the policy tells me.' Here, the psychosocial issues centre on the incompatibility of *being too busy* and not having to worry about undertaking standard precautions or adhering to the policy. However, the practitioner's thinking is unsound as a result of their failing to recognise that adopting standard precautions and adhering to the policy are related to caring for the patient.

➤ **In the case of an administrator:** This person believes that hand hygiene is not important because they do not make physical contact with patients or clients. Here, the psychosocial issues centre on the incompatibility of the administrator believing that hand hygiene is not necessary and justifying this with the excuse that physical contact with patients or clients is not a part of their role. However, the administrator's thinking is unsound because of their belief that physical contact between individuals is not necessary for cross infection to occur.

REFLECTION EXERCISE 1.2

Take some time to think about your own infection control practice. It is important that you are absolutely honest and do not make excuses.

Ask yourself 'How good am I at preventing cross infection?' Write down your feelings and then reflect upon them using the following template:

Subjective reflection process

Who: Who else can support my assumptions regarding my ability to reduce the risk of cross infection?

What: What research/evidence can I provide that will support my assumptions?

When: When am I most at risk of committing infection control violations?

Where: Where does my working environment contribute to my committing infection control violations?

How: How can I prevent myself from committing infection control violations?

Why: Why should I care if I commit infection control violations or not?

Critical reflection process

NB: This part requires you to look at your list of feelings drawn from the subjective reflection process above, and to challenge those feelings.

Who Says So? For example:

- How do I know that my subjective reflections above are valid, reliable and correct?
- If I were to discuss my subjective reflections above with a colleague, would their conclusions be different to mine?
- If I commit infection control violations, where do I stand ethically, morally and legally?
- If I commit infection control violations could I be breaching another person's human rights? Could I be in contravention of health and safety legislation? Could I be in contravention of any codes of conduct or prescriptive rules to which I am subject?
- Is it really the working environment that contributes to my committing infection control violations or is blaming the environment simply an excuse for my own failings?

Then ask yourself (make a list if you like, as it may aid you in clarifying your thinking):

- What have I done in the past that might have served to reduce the spread of healthcare-acquired infections?
- What have I done in the past that could have increased the risk of spreading healthcare-acquired infections to myself and others?

If you decide that you have never done anything to increase the risk of healthcare-acquired infections then you are probably not being honest. The simple fact that you are human and fallible increases the risk of you committing infection control violations. (Extracts from Elliott in Jasper 2006.)

In consideration of non-adherence to infection control practices in the form of failing to adopt standard precautions or follow prescriptive rules, it would be unjust to single out any particular individual, role, profession or gender. To do so would be unprofessional. Yet this is exactly what many health and social care professionals do. They attribute non-adherence and cross-infection rates to every other individual or profession with the exception of the person making the accusation.

REFLECTION EXERCISE 1.3

Who do you think is responsible for increasing rates of cross infection?

What kinds of objects do you carry on your person that could constitute an infection risk? Compare your list with List 1.2.

Having thought about the two questions above, what will you do in the future?

LIST 1.2 OBJECTS CARRIED ON THE PERSON THAT CAN CONSTITUTE A CROSS-INFECTION RISK

1 Scissors or forceps in pockets
   Reflection points:
   - What do you use these for?
   - When did you last clean them?
   - What did you clean them with?
   - What do you also carry in the pocket in which you carry the scissors?

2 Surgical tape in pockets
   Reflection points:
   - Why do you carry the tape?
   - How long has the roll of tape been in your pocket?
   - What do you use the tape for?
   - When you look at the roll of tape how clean does it appear?

3 Paper tissues in pockets
   Reflection points:
   - What have you used the tissues for?
   - When you have used a tissue do you put it back in your pocket?
   - What do you also carry in your pockets with these tissues? This is particularly important if you put used tissues back in your pocket.
   - If you have used the tissues to sneeze into or to wipe your nose, do you adopt hand hygiene afterwards?

4 Badges, stethoscopes, tourniquets
   Reflection points:
   - When were these last cleaned?
   - When you look at them, how clean do they appear?
   - When not in use, where do you keep them?
   - If you keep them in a pocket, what else is in the pocket?

5 Uniforms, work clothing, ties
   Reflection points:
   - When were the ties and jackets last cleaned?

- Once you've removed your work clothing, where do you keep/place it prior to washing?
- How often do you change uniforms?

NB: All of the above are potential sources of cross infection. They should be perceived as examples and are not mutually exclusive.

Such accusations are prejudicial, discriminatory and unethical because in reality non-adherence is common among a large proportion of those involved in the provision of healthcare. There can be no doubt that cross infection through such non-adherence is of significant concern where the health, safety and welfare of patients and clients are concerned. Despite this, and a research base of some 200 years (Elliott 2003), cross infection, as a result of non-adherence to standard precautions and prescriptive rules, continues to have an impact upon the lives of individuals. Further, although many of those involved in health and social care clearly understand the need for safe infection control practice, they regularly fail to behave in ways that would serve to reduce the risks of healthcare-acquired infections. For example:

➤ travelling home in work clothing and stopping off to go shopping;
➤ changing out of work clothing at home and placing it in the same container as other non-work-related clothing for laundering;
➤ leaving the operating theatre environment wearing a white coat over their tunic and trousers in the belief that this will reduce the risk of cross infection;
➤ failing to change disposable aprons between patients or failing to change uniforms on a daily basis because they were not visibly contaminated;
➤ failing to undertake appropriate hand hygiene between clean/dirty tasks or if hand hygiene is undertaken, failing to adhere to the hand hygiene process (*see* List 1.3).

LIST 1.3 HAND HYGIENE PROCESS (ELLIOTT 2003)

There are six stages within the hand hygiene process. The omission of any stage within the process or a simple failure to follow the process will serve to increase the risk of infecting yourself or cross infecting others.

Stage 1 – It is vital that you recognise the need to undertake hand hygiene. This is probably the most important stage within the process because if you fail to recognise situations where you need to adopt formal hand hygiene, as opposed to using hand cleansing rubs/gels, then the remainder of the process will at worst not occur and at best occur intermittently. Either way the risk of cross infection will be increased.

Stage 2 – It is important that you wet all areas to be washed thoroughly with running water. Failure do this may lead to you experiencing skin problems because some cleansing agents can cause irritation of the skin if applied prior to wetting the areas to be washed. The rule being always read the manufacturer's recommendations.

Stage 3 – It is important that you always apply an appropriate cleansing agent to the areas for washing. The type of agent will be determined by the nature of the intended intervention:
- invasive/surgical
- antiseptic
- social.

It is not necessary to apply excessive amounts of the cleansing solution and the manufacturer's recommendations should always be followed.

Stage 4 – It is important that when washing the areas to be cleansed/decontaminated, an approved method and time period are adhered to:
- invasive/surgical: minimum 2 minutes – hands, wrists and up to the elbow;
- antiseptic: minimum 30 seconds – hands, wrists and up to mid-forearm;
- social: minimum 15 seconds – hands and wrists.

Stage 5 – It is important that you rinse all the areas washed, until all trace of the cleansing agent has gone. Failure to do this may lead to skin irritation resulting from traces of the cleansing agent being left on your skin. In addition, where traces of the cleansing agent are left on the skin this may serve to facilitate bacterial re-colonisation.

Stage 6 – It is important to thoroughly dry all of the areas washed, using:
- sterile hand towels for invasive/surgical interventions;
- sterile or disposable hand towels depending upon the nature of the intervention;
- disposable hand towels or hot air blowers for social interventions.

NB:
1   When using hand towels, a sufficient number must be used to ensure that the areas washed are completely dry. Failure to do this will mean that the areas you have washed will still be damp/moist and as such bacterial re-colonisation will be facilitated.
2   Hot air blowers are not appropriate for positioning in any clinical environment.

However, if your workplace does contain hot air blowers, they should be regularly cleaned and maintained both inside and out. The next time you come across a hot air blower in an environment where you have been working, have a look at the inlet and outlet grills where air is drawn in and blown out. Ask yourself: 'What do I see and will it be likely to re-contaminate the areas that I have just so meticulously cleaned?' If you are concerned by your answer to the first question, and 'Yes' is your answer to the second question, do not just walk away; report it.

Psychosocial factors that will serve to facilitate failure to undertake all or some of the above stages are:
- dissonance effects
- cognitively economic thinking
- egocentric attitudes
- complacency
- fatigue
- stress
- low morale
- excessive work load
- unrealistic optimism
- task-orientated perspective
- the 'It will not happen to me' syndrome
- adopting a biomedical approach.

Such behaviour has ethical, moral and legal implications in terms of breaching the individual's human rights (*see* List 1.4) as well as international health and safety law (Taylor 2002), because such laws are intended to reflect the principle that each individual should take all reasonable steps to ensure the health, safety and welfare of others. In addition, those health and social care professionals who fail to undertake appropriate infection control practices are placing little value upon the ethics and morality of what they do (Seedhouse 1998), and may be in contravention of their employer's prescriptive rules and any professional code of conduct to which they are subject.

LIST 1.4 INFECTION CONTROL VIOLATIONS AND
HUMAN RIGHTS INFRINGEMENTS

Clarifying Statement: The articles referred to below are drawn from the above source and relate to the European Human Rights Act 1998 presented within

Wilkinson and Caulfield (2001). Within the Act each human right is referred to as an 'Article'. This should not be confused with an article that may be published in an academic journal.

Article 1 – Obligations to secure rights and freedoms: Every individual has the right to expect to be kept safe from cross infection by health and social care professionals. If a health and social care professional fails to adopt appropriate standard precautions and thus increases the risk of cross infection, a colleague, patient or client might argue that their human rights have been infringed.

Article 2 – Right to life: Every individual has the right to have their life protected. If an individual involved in the provision of healthcare knows they should undertake appropriate hand hygiene but fails to do so, then this may be deemed as an intentional act of omission, which could impact upon a patient or client's life in terms of their general health and wellbeing, and their ability to carry out normal activities of daily living (Roper, Logan and Tierney 2000) or even result in their death. Therefore, under such circumstances, if a health or social care professional fails to undertake hand hygiene in accordance with the hand hygiene process (*see* List 1.3), a patient or client might argue that their human rights have been infringed.

Article 3 – Prohibition of torture: Individuals have a right not to experience pain and suffering or feel degraded as a result of an act of omission on the part of health and social care professionals. An act of omission in this case would be where an infection control violation occurs, which leads to a patient or client contracting a healthcare-acquired infection. As a consequence of contracting a healthcare-acquired infection, a patient or client experiences pain and suffering, resulting in a loss of self-esteem, which in turn leads to a sense of feeling degraded as a person. In such a situation, a patient or client may argue that their human rights have been infringed. It is important to remember that torture may be Physical (the experience of physiological pain), Psychological (the experience of emotional distress, anxiety or stress) or Social (the experience of enforced isolation or of being ostracised).

Article 5 – Right to liberty and security: Patients and clients have a right to liberty in the sense that having voluntarily entered and consented to treatment within a healthcare establishment they should not be forced to remain within that establishment any longer than necessary. If a patient or client is forced to remain within a healthcare establishment longer than necessary as a result of infection control violations committed by health and social care professionals, leading to the contracting of a healthcare-acquired infection, it might be presupposed that their liberty has been restricted through no fault of their own.

In such a situation, a patient or client might argue that their human rights have been infringed.

Article 10 – Freedom of expression: Every individual has the right of expression with regard to questioning or challenging the treatment they receive, the quality of the care they are provided with and any decisions that are made regarding their future health and wellbeing by health and social care professionals. Should a patient or client observe an infection control violation, for example in the form of a health or social care professional failing to change a disposable apron appropriately or failing to adopt appropriate hand hygiene, then they would have the right to question or challenge the professional's behaviour. In such a situation, if their right to question or challenge were denied or refused, a patient or client might argue that their human rights have been infringed, as such acts of omission would serve to increase the risk of cross infection leading to the patient or client contracting a healthcare-acquired infection.

Article 11 – Prohibition of discrimination: Where an individual questions and challenges the behaviour of a health or social care professional and as a result of such experiences ridicule, defamatory statements or professional neglect, they may feel discriminated against. In such a situation a patient or client might argue that their human rights have been infringed. In addition, if such were to occur then a patient or client might argue that their human rights have been further infringed under Articles 2, 3 and 5 as a result of any potential pain, suffering or sense of humiliation they might experience leading to an impact upon their right to life and liberty.

NB: The above-listed Articles should not be perceived as being mutually exclusive, but as offering a perspective.

Historically, knowledge of infection control and standard precautions is by no means new. The ancient Egyptians, Greeks and Romans developed an understanding of both cross infection and the need for appropriate hygiene (Trueman 2002). Around 1822 Labarraque discovered a link between hand hygiene and cross infection and some 25 years later Semmelweis during the mid-1800s achieved a reduction in cross-infection rates through the application of hand hygiene (Weinstein 2004). Even during the Crimean War (1854–56), Florence Nightingale recognised the need for good hygiene (infection-control practices) in the form of regular changes of bed linen, adequate ventilation, regular emptying of chamber pots and regular scrubbing of the floors and walls (Harvard University Library), yet within our modern global society we are still unable to resolve the problems of cross infection as a result of non-adherence to standard precautions. Why is this? It is because we are all incessant risk-takers. When such risk-taking is combined with the 'It will not happen to me' syndrome (Elliott 2003) it will inevitably result in increased levels of non-adherence to standard precautions. Further, such risk-taking will be enhanced if the health or social care professional believes that they are not responsible for such cross infection.

Such risk-taking, non-adherence and questionable beliefs have particular relevance for patients or clients seeking healthcare intervention with regard to their expectations that such interventions will both promote their future health and wellbeing and their ability to carry out normal activities of daily living (Roper, Logan and Tierney 2000). Yet currently, such expectations fail to be fulfilled on a consistent basis with many patients and clients contracting what can be described as *an added extra*. Such added extras include a variety of healthcare-acquired infections, which result in physical, psychological and social injury for the individuals concerned.

REFLECTION EXERCISE 1.4

Consider what types of physical, psychological and social injury a patient or client of yours experienced as a result of contracting an added extra in the form of a healthcare-acquired infection.

You may find it useful to make a list for each type of injury. Once you have completed your list compare it with Table 1.1.

To what degree do you think you were responsible for causing such physical, psychological and social injury?

The three types of injury shown in Table 1.1 may result from contracting a healthcare-acquired infection.

TABLE 1.1 Examples of physical, psychological and social injury

Physical	Psychological	Social
Wounds	Anxiety	Loss of independence
Body scarring	Distress	Loss of social networks
Loss of mobility	Anger	Isolation
Physiological pain	Emotional pain	Pain resulting from loss of identity
Unpleasant odours	Complacency	
Sleep deprivation	Demotivation	Loss of income

(continued)

Physical	Psychological	Social
Reduced communication	Demoralisation	Loss of social status
Non-compliance	Paranoia	Stereotyping
Negative perception of body image	Mood swings	Distrust
	Boredom	Labelling
Altered states of consciousness	Low self-esteem	Sleep deprivation
	Depression	Institutionalisation
	Loss of identity	Disorientation
	Negative memories	Reduced communication
	Stress	Reduced socialisation
	Mental health problems	Reactive behaviour related to healthcare needs
	Emotional outbursts	
		Unpleasant odours
		Social withdrawal
		Non-compliance to social norms

NB: The above should not be seen as mutually exclusive, but as providing examples.

With regard to such physical, psychological and social injury, although the consequences may have little, if any effect upon health and social care professionals, the effects can be devastating and life-long for the individual, their relatives and friends. It is unacceptable that individuals seeking help from those who profess to care should be subject to dangers resulting from risk-taking behaviours in the form of non-adherence to standard precautions (*see* List 1.1). It would seem that where the prevention of healthcare-acquired infections is concerned, many health and social care professionals – irrespective of their appointment, profession or role – have failed those they owe their allegiance to and those they profess to care about most: the patients and clients.

Despite this, there have been initiatives aimed at reducing cross infection, which have led to some success in reducing healthcare-acquired infections in the short and medium term. However, success in reducing healthcare-acquired infections should not be seen as conclusive evidence of behavioural change where improved adherence to standard precautions is concerned. Making such a link would be very tenuous as any reduction in the rates of healthcare-acquired infections might have been the result of random chance or something the recipient of healthcare might have done themselves. It may have had nothing to do with anything the health or social care professional did or did not do.

Source →	Stimulus →	Assumed response →	Rationale →	Actual response →	Rationale
Manager →	Instigation of a prescriptive rule. →	Consistent and unchallenged adherence. →	Because of who I am. →	Rejection, resentment and non-adherence. →	No time, something else to do and what's in it for me?
Lecturer →	Delivery of information. →	Will accept and believe what I say. →	Because I am knowledgeable and know what I am talking about. →	Ridicule and boredom; disregard of delivered information. →	Who says you know what you are talking about?
Trainer →	Practical instruction and having a go. →	They have carried out the procedure. →	I have watched them; they are therefore competent. →	OK, they have watched me; now I am on my own I will do it my way. →	My colleagues do it my way; it has always been done the way I do it, so why change?

FIGURE 1.1 Stimulus/response approach.

What initiatives have served to reduce the spread of healthcare-acquired infections within your working area? How have they served to reduce healthcare-acquired infections occurring within that area?

If your answer is 'none' then what implications does this have with regard to your safety and the safety of others?

Despite initiatives such as regular education and training, enforced prescriptive rules, the provision of hand cleansing rubs/gels (which, contrary to the beliefs of some, are not an absolute substitute for formal hand hygiene (*see* List 1.3)), audit processes, media campaigns, financial infusions or the appointment of modern matrons, there is to date no clear evidence to indicate that safe infection control practice has been achieved on a consistent long-term basis.

In the case of education, as far back as 1988, Williams and Buckles identified no clear correlation between what an individual knows and the way they behave where adherence to safe infection control practice is concerned. Yet there continues to be heavy reliance placed upon what might be described as the Stimulus-Response (S and R) approach (Atkinson *et al.* 2000) (*see* Figure 1.1) where there is an irrational belief among some people that the more we tell health and social care professionals they must do something (the stimulus) the more they will consistently adhere (response). Such a belief is particularly inherent among many within health service management, higher education and healthcare provider training departments. For example, managers assume that by instigating a prescriptive rule it will be successful; lecturers assume that because they say something is so it will be followed; or trainers who assume that practical instruction/experience will lead to safe practice. None of these assumptions will ensure consistent adherence to anything. Why is this? Because in many cases all three groups fail to incorporate psychological and social elements into what they wish to achieve.

CONCLUSION

In this first chapter, it has been my intention to stimulate both your thinking about the psychosocial issues involved in infection control and your own and others' infection control behaviour.

REFERENCES

Atkinson RL, Atkinson RC, Smith E, *et al. Hilgard's Introduction to Psychology*. 13th ed. London: Harcourt College; 2000.

Elliott P. Recognising the psychosocial issues involved in hand hygiene. *J R Soc Health.* 2003; **123**(2): 88–94.

Elliott P. Understanding clinical supervision: a health psychology orientated process of person-centred development. In: Jasper M, editor. *Vital Notes for Nurses: professional development, reflection and decision making.* Oxford: Blackwell; 2006.

Harvard University Library Open Collections Program: Contagion. *Florence Nightingale, 1820–1910.* Available at: http://ocp.hul.harvard.edu/contagion/nightingale.html (accessed 25 Nov 2008).

Lawton R, Parker D. Procedures and the professional: the case of the British NHS. *Soc Sci Med.* 1999; **48**: 353–61.

Reason J, Parker D, Lawton R. Organisational controls and safety: the varieties of role-related behaviour. *J Occup Organ Psychol.* 1998; **71**: 289–304.

Roper N, Logan W, Tierney A. *The Roper-Logan-Tierney Model of Nursing: based on activities of living.* London: Churchill Livingstone; 2000.

Seedhouse D. *Ethics: the heart of healthcare.* 2nd ed. Chichester: John Wiley and Sons; 1998.

Taylor A. Global governance, international health law and WHO: looking towards the future. *Bull World Health Organ.* 2002; **80**(12): 975–80.

Trueman C. *Medicine in Ancient Rome.* Sackville School, East Grinstead, UK; 2002. Available at: www.historylearningsite.co.uk/medicine_in_ancient_rome.htm (accessed 25 Nov 2008).

Weinstein R. Hand hygiene: of reason and ritual. *Ann Intern Med.* 2004; **141**(1): 65–6.

Wilkinson R, Caulfield H. *The Human Rights Act: a practical guide for nurses.* Chichester: John Wiley; 2001.

Williams E, Buckles A. A lack of motivation. *Nurs Times (Journal of Infection Control Nursing).* 1988; **84**(22): 63–4.

INTRODUCTION

Lynn Parker and I first met in 2002 at the Infection Control Nurses Association International Conference. During our various conversations both at the conference and subsequently, I have developed much respect for Lynn's considerable expertise and knowledge within the context of infection control. Lynn is the co-founder of Healthcare A2Z, which aims to provide practical information, education and communication solutions for health and social care professionals.

Although Lynn has included a number of reflection exercises throughout this chapter, you may find it useful to reflect upon how this information impacts upon your own infection control practice.

CHAPTER 2

Perspectives from the clinical setting

Lynn Parker

INTRODUCTION

Often considered to be one of the Cinderella services of the NHS, the practice of infection, prevention and control has now come under the spotlight from government, media and the general public. Not only are they concerned with healthcare associated infections (HCAI), but also there is a fear of bioterrorism with diseases such as smallpox, anthrax or botulism. International outbreaks of severe acute respiratory syndrome (SARS) also give concerns as to when the next influenza pandemic will be.

This chapter refers to the current legislative framework around infection prevention and control. It discusses the role of the infection control nurse for implementing change and the evidence base for clinical practice.

LEGISLATION AND GUIDANCE

HCAI were identified in the Chief Medical Officer's Infectious Diseases Strategy for England, *Getting Ahead of the Curve* (Department of Health 2002). The intention was to bring infection control issues into the mainstream service area of improvement. To this end, numerous guidance and circulars have been published since 1998 with key documents including:

➤ the Standing Medical Advisory Committee report on antimicrobial resistance (1998);

➤ controls assurance standard on infection control produced in 1999 and revised in 2004, which provides a checklist of measures for acute hospitals to manage the environment and to have structures and processes in place for an effective infection control team (National Health Service Executive 2001);

➤ the Health Service circular issued in 2000 setting out the requirements for the effective decontamination of medical devices (Department of Health 2000);

➤ the National Audit Report into the control of hospital-acquired infection in Acute Trusts in England in 2000 (National Audit Office 2000), which was repeated four years later (National Audit Office 2004);

➤ evidence-based guidelines published in 2001 on the prevention and control of hospital-acquired infection (Pratt *et al.* 2001);

➤ mandatory surveillance scheme in England for serious (bloodstream) infections caused by *Staphylococcus aureus* including methicillin-resistant *Staphylococcus aureus* (MRSA) in 2001 (Department of Health 2003a);

➤ evidence-based guidelines published in 2003 on the prevention of healthcare associated infection in primary and community care settings (Pellowe *et al.* 2003);

➤ guidance by the Medicines and Healthcare products Regulatory Agency (MHRA) on the decontamination of medical devices (Medicines and Healthcare Products Regulatory Agency 2003);

➤ two performance management indicators related to HCAI in the Star Ratings system for acute hospital NHS Trusts in England (The Commission for Health Improvement 2003);

➤ the Chief Medical Officer's report, *Winning Ways*, which sets out seven areas of action to be taken on HCAI and antimicrobial resistance (Department of Health 2003b);

➤ the Department of Health report on saving lives, which provided a delivery programme to reduce healthcare-associated infections (Department of Health 2005);

➤ a step-by-step framework for safe, clean care, with tools and techniques to audit clinical practice was produced to prevent the spread of infection (Department of Health 2006a);

➤ the Health Act 2006 included a code of practice, which states the duties that an NHS organisation has to follow to prevent and control HCAI (Department of Health 2006b).

With such a number of initiatives from the government, increasing demands have been placed upon infection control teams and their allocated resources. This is compounded by other NHS initiatives, such as increased throughput of patients and trolley-waits in emergency departments, which result in higher bed-occupancy rates above the target of 82% for 2003–04 (National Audit Office 2004). In addition, the lack of suitable isolation facilities, partial-compliance to screening programmes on admission for MRSA colonisation policies, frequent movement of patients between hospitals, wards and departments, and insufficient beds to separate elective and trauma patients – particularly in orthopaedic and vascular surgery – all increase the difficulty of achieving the practice of prevention and control of infection.

Since devolution in 1999 there have been variations in the approach to HCAI between the four countries of the UK (England, Scotland, Wales and Northern Ireland) with each setting their own strategy and emphasis relevant to their individual health needs. All the strategies from the four countries address the need for surveillance, education, clinical standards of practice and improvement of antimicrobial prescribing.

REFLECTION EXERCISE 2.1

Consider the 11 duties listed in the Health Code 2006 (Department of Health 2006b). How would they apply to your area of clinical practice?

THE CHANGING ROLE OF THE INFECTION CONTROL NURSE: EXPERT DATA COLLECTOR OR INTERVENTIONIST?

What was once a solitary role for infection control nurses (ICNs) working on their own in an acute general hospital has now at the beginning of the 21st century widened to that of a team approach, where different skills in surveillance, audit and clinical practice are required. The role now encompasses prevention as well as controlling infections, and post holders work in a variety of settings including acute, community, public health and the management of communicable diseases. Role development for individual nurses has moved from that of 'on the job' training, which was provided by the infection control doctor, to a dedicated and structured educational framework to Masters and Doctorate levels specifically in infection control. Not only can nurses achieve specialist practitioner status, but they can also attain consultant nurse posts in the hospital and community and so provide a career pathway within the speciality. Role development through education starts with role identification, then moves through novice practitioner to becoming a change agent and finally arriving at an advisory/consultancy role (Horton and Parker 2002).

Infection prevention and control is one of the few specialist roles that carries organisational and population-wide responsibility. As such, one of the aims of infection control nurses is to achieve compliance with good infection control practices by all healthcare workers and for them to accept their own responsibilities regarding the infections that their patients acquire.

REFLECTION EXERCISE 2.2

Compare the job descriptions and role definitions of infection control practitioners in a variety of settings and at different levels within an organisation.
● Discuss the differences and similarities between the roles.
● Consider the educational training required to be competent in the different roles.
● Do the roles reflect the core competencies for infection control nurses developed by the Infection Control Nurses Association (Tew *et al.* 2002)?

Initiating and implementing change can be difficult to achieve and change is not something that can be done quickly. Infection control nurses need to be aware of the strategies for achieving change, including factors that can help and those that hinder. Factors that assist change include:
➤ initial and continuing education of staff to increase their awareness and understanding;
➤ clear procedures and protocols;
➤ consistent and clear communications;
➤ availability of resources;
➤ role models;
➤ creating a culture that values safe practice.

Factors that hinder or prevent change include:
➤ inappropriate perceptions of the risk involved in work practices;
➤ lack of resources;
➤ poor levels of knowledge and motivation;
➤ poor role models;
➤ the 'it won't happen to me' syndrome.

Change also affects ICNs in their own roles. This has been especially evident over the past five years with the increased requirements of mandatory surveillance, audit and external inspections resulting in a mismatch between the expectations placed upon the infection control team and the resources of staff, time and money allocated to them. With the expansion of infection control teams and the changing focus of the role, there is a need for ICNs to educate themselves about the changing healthcare environment and to actively anticipate change before it is imposed by external forces.

ICNs might identify themselves with the characters in *Who Moved My Cheese?* (Johnson 1998). A story of mice and men caught in a maze, it describes the stresses involved in change and suggests strategies that can be taken to manage it. The points to remember from the story are that:

➤ change happens (they keep moving the cheese);
➤ anticipate change (get ready for the cheese to move);
➤ monitor change (smell the cheese often so you know when it's getting old);
➤ adapt to change quickly (the quicker you let go of old cheese, the sooner you'll find new cheese to enjoy);
➤ change: enjoy it and be ready to do it again (because they keep moving the cheese).

The latest National Audit Office report for England and Wales (National Audit Office 2004) states that infections are still perceived as the problem for infection control teams. Barriers to good practice still remain and change needs to be achieved in education and training for all healthcare staff to gain compliance in hand hygiene, clinical practices such as catheter care and aseptic technique, antibiotic prescribing and hospital cleanliness.

Implementing the latest government guidance, *Winning Ways* (Department of Health 2003b) will place increasing demands upon infection control teams, despite it being aimed at all NHS staff. To support such guidance there has been the publication of frameworks and audit tools from the Department of Health in England, which organisations can use as a means to evaluate the level of compliance and identify areas of practice for improvement (Department of Health 2005, 2006a). By signing up to participate in these programmes, organisations will be perceived as complying to the new Health Code (Department of Health 2006b) by the Healthcare Commission.

In Scotland, the approach has been to introduce 'model policies,' which healthcare organisations can use and adapt to local needs and issues (Health Protection Scotland 2006). These have been supported by the encouragement of participation in educational programmes, such as the 'cleanliness champions' (NHS Education for Scotland 2003). Both Wales and Northern Ireland have produced strategic guidance stating how the prevention and control of HCAI can be achieved (DHSSPSNI 2006; Welsh Assembly 2004).

EVIDENCE-BASED PRACTICE (CORE PROCESSES AND ACTIVITIES OF INFECTION CONTROL)

The Centre for Evidence-Based Nursing website states that evidence-based nursing is 'the process by which nurses make clinical decisions using the best available research evidence, their clinical expertise and patient preferences in the context of available resources' (Dicenso, Cullum and Ciliska 1998, p. 38).

With the advance of technology and the use of the Internet, it has never been easier to access information, but what is questionable is the quality of the information accessed. Many resources are available through databases such as Medline and the Cochrane Library, evidence-based journals, the National Library for Health (NLH) and guidance from the National Institute for Clinical Excellence (NICE). Whilst it is possible to access much information on the Internet it is worthwhile remembering the maxim of 'rubbish in, equals rubbish out.' Befriending a librarian is always worthwhile as they can teach you to find material, filter out the best evidence and navigate the Internet effectively and quickly.

Infections are caused by multiple factors and according to Horton and Parker (2002) include:

➤ patient risk factors: underlying illness, weakened immunity;
➤ external risk factors: invasive devices that breach normal defence mechanisms;
➤ organisation risk factors: high bed occupancy, lack of isolation, movement of patients in the system, poor staffing levels;
➤ behavioural risk factors: poor compliance to policies, change of practice to reflect research;
➤ structural risk factors: lack of isolation rooms, inadequate hand wash facilities;
➤ environmental risk factors: cleanliness of the environment, instruments and equipment used;
➤ national risk factors: inappropriate use of antibiotics in medicine and agriculture.

Whilst the focus and amount of time allocated to each of the above components of an infection, prevention and control programme have varied between countries throughout the world, it is still agreed that if all the elements are put into practice they will reduce the incidence of infection by 15%. Some specialists state that this could even be as high as 30% (Department of Health 2003b; Horton and Parker 2002; National Audit Office 2004).

Kitson's (1995) description of clinical effectiveness as 'doing the right thing' and 'doing the thing right' suggests a level of knowledge that enables healthcare practitioners to 'do it right' and evaluate the care that they deliver to patients. There are now evidence-based guidelines for both the acute and the primary and community sectors on which to base local policies (Pellowe *et al.* 2003; Pratt *et al.* 2001). Since the publication of these two papers, infection control teams have struggled with implementing these guidelines in local practice.

The guidelines are methodically-developed broad principles of good practice. Evidence was taken from systematic reviews and meta-analyses, experimental studies, consensus papers, expert opinion and national and international guideline recommendations. This evidence was then synthesised and graded into the following three categories:

➤ Category 1: generally consistent findings in a range of evidence derived from a majority of acceptable studies;
➤ Category 2: evidence based on a single acceptable study, or a weak or inconsistent finding in multiple acceptable studies;
➤ Category 3: limited scientific evidence that does not meet all the criteria of 'acceptable studies' or an absence of directly applicable studies of good quality, including published expert opinion derived from systematically retrieved and appraised professional, national and international guidelines.

Guidelines for acute hospitals (Pratt *et al.* 2001) provided evidence for:
➤ Standard principles for preventing hospital-acquired infections:
  — hospital environmental hygiene;
  — hand hygiene;
  — the use of personal protective equipment;
  — the use and disposal of sharps.
➤ Guidelines for preventing infections associated with the use of short-term indwelling urethral catheters in acute care:
  — assessing the need for catheterisation;
  — selection of catheter type;
  — aseptic catheter insertion;
  — catheter maintenance.
➤ Guidelines for preventing infections associated with the insertion and maintenance of central venous catheters:
  — selection of catheter type;
  — selection of catheter insertion site;
  — aseptic technique during catheter insertion;
  — cutaneous antisepsis;

— catheter and catheter site care;
— catheter replacement strategies;
— antibiotic prophylaxis.

Guidelines for primary and community care (Pellowe *et al.* 2003) provided evidence for:

➤ Standard principles:
  — hand hygiene;
  — the use of personal protective equipment;
  — the safe use and disposal of sharps;
  — education of patients, their carers and healthcare personnel.
➤ Care of patients with long-term urinary catheters:
  — education of patients, their carers and healthcare personnel;
  — assessing the need for catheterisation;
  — selection of catheter drainage options;
  — catheter insertion;
  — catheter maintenance.
➤ Care during enteral feeding:
  — education of patients, their carers and healthcare personnel;
  — preparation and storage of feeds;
  — administration of feeds;
  — care of insertion site and enteral feeding tube.
➤ Care of patients with central venous catheters:
  — education of patients, their carers and healthcare personnel;
  — general asepsis;
  — catheter site care;
  — general principles for catheter management.

Both sets of guidelines recognise the lack of evidence on which current practice is based and the need for further research.

Examples of using the guidelines to effect change in clinical practice are available. Duncanson and Heath (2003) showed that by working with a multi-disciplinary team and using a quality improvement programme they could change clinical practice. Taking the guideline on the use of short-term urinary catheterisation, through the use of an audit and surveillance framework they improved the knowledge and practice of nurses, documentation and change in practice.

Along with providing a knowledge base from which practitioners can deliver safe care, infection control nurses often use the power of persuasion. Raven and Haley (1982) described six categories of power used to influence the change in behaviour of nurses who repeatedly break technique and exposed patients to a high risk of infection by not following correct infection control procedures. The six categories of power were:

1   Coercive power: warning of possible disciplinary action or dismissal;
2   Reward: reminding of the influence carried by the ICN, which could be advantageous to the nurse's future;
3   Legitimate: emphasising the ICN's position and the nurse's obligation to comply;
4   Referent: emphasising that proper procedures are followed by other nurses in the hospital;
5   Expert: emphasising the ICN's own expertise regarding infection control procedures;
6   Information: indicating the reason for infection control techniques through evidence, research and available literature.

Those that gained the majority support were information, expert and referent powers (Horton and Parker 2002).

Infection control teams need to be adequately resourced to achieve all that is required of them. The time spent building relationships with clinical managers, finance directors, suppliers, educationalists and other colleagues can affect the amount of active participation from colleagues in all areas of the organisation in preventing infections in patients.

REFLECTION EXERCISE 2.3

Consider an area of clinical practice where you have implemented or influenced change.
- Who did you need to involve?
- What categories of power did you use?

OUTDATED INFECTION CONTROL PRACTICES

Even though evidence-based practice is promoted to colleagues in a variety of clinical settings, there are a number of infection control practices that could be described as ritualistic, based on the current available evidence (Pirwitz and Manian 1997).

There is considerable unwillingness to 'let go' of old practices. Studies in the USA show that a proportion of infection control practitioners were reluctant to remove certain practices from their own clinical areas (Jackson 1999).

In 1997 Pirwitz and Manian identified the following outdated infection control practices considered to be infection control rituals which no longer should be followed but which healthcare staff continue to implement:

- everything in the room of a patient placed in isolation should be considered contaminated and discarded or disinfected when the patient is discharged;
- use of sterile linen for neutropenic patients;
- double-bagging of waste and soiled linen from isolation rooms;
- use of disposable dishes or trays for patients in isolation;
- use of 'tacky mats' in the operating room and the entrances of high dependency units;
- dedicated equipment for HIV patients;
- changing intravenous tubing every 24 hours;
- changing ventilator tubing every 24–48 hours.

> (Pirwitz and Manian 1997 (this reference applies to all the above bullet points).)

Current evidence-based guidelines provide a platform for further research on the efficacy of clinical practices to prevent HCAI. The strength of current evidence is often limited and the authors of the guidelines called for further research (Manangan *et al.* 2001; Pellowe *et al.* 2003; Pratt *et al.* 2001). There are still outdated practices being performed both in hospitals and other healthcare institutions. Through the use of audits such practices can be identified and changes made. A recent audit of a GP surgery identified the use of unsterilised equipment and resulted in the suspension of a nurse and the recalling and counselling of patients affected (Cooper 2003).

What is important is that once a need for change has been identified, it can be effected and monitored, and compliance achieved through ongoing education and training for all staff.

CONCLUSION

Whilst there is a legislative framework to guide the practice of infection prevention and control, increasing demands to achieve government targets present competing aims for NHS trusts in England (National Audit Office 2004). The role change of ICNs and the diverse nature of healthcare in which it is practised make it a specialisation with organisational and population-wide responsibilities. Within each nursing generation there is a call that practice is based on the best available evidence. To achieve such an aim it is important that ICNs learn to recognise change, embrace it and use it to improve clinical practice.

REFERENCES

Cooper K. Bad practice discovered by infection control nurse. *Nurs Stand.* 2003; **17**(44): 8.

Department of Health. Decontamination of medical devices. *Health Service Circular* (HSC 2000/032). London: Department of Health; 2000.

Department of Health. Getting ahead of the curve: a strategy for combating infectious diseases. *A Report by the Chief Medical Officer.* London: Department of Health; 2002.

Department of Health. Surveillance of healthcare associated infections. *Professional Letter, Chief Medical Officer:* PLCMO (2003) 04. London: Department of Health; 2003a.

Department of Health. Winning ways: working together to reduce healthcare associated infection in England. *Report from the Chief Medical Officer.* London: Department of Health; 2003b.

Department of Health. *Saving Lives: a delivery programme to reduce healthcare-associated infection including MRSA.* London: Department of Health; 2005.

Department of Health. *Essential Steps to Safe, Clean Care: preventing the spread of infection.* London: Department of Health; 2006a.

Department of Health. *The Health Act 2006: code of practice for the prevention and control of healthcare associated infections.* London: Department of Health; 2006b.

Department of Health Standing Medical Advisory Committee Sub-Group on Antimicrobial Resistance. *The Path of Least Resistance: summary and recommendations.* London: Department of Health; 1998.

DHSSPSNI 2006. *Changing the Culture: an action plan for the prevention and control of healthcare associated infections in Northern Ireland 2006/2009.* Available at: www. dhsspsni.gov.uk/hcai_action_plan.pdf (accessed 25 Nov 2008).

Dicenso A, Cullum N, Ciliska D. Implementing evidence-based nursing: some misconceptions. *Evid Based Nurs.* 1998; **1**(2): 38–40.

Duncanson V, Heath T. Developing effective clinical practice: 'making it harder to do it wrong, making it easier to do it right.' *Br J Infect Control.* 2003; **4**(5): 28–33.

Health Protection Scotland 2006. *Model Infection Control Policies.* Available at: www.hps. scot.nhs.uk/haiic/ic/modelinfectioncontrolpolicies.aspx (accessed 25 Nov 2008).

Horton R, Parker L. *Informed Infection Control Practice.* 2nd ed. New York: Churchill Livingstone; 2002.

Jackson MM. The healthcare marketplace in the next millennium and nurses' roles in infection prevention and control. *Nurs Clin North Am.* 1999; **34**(2): 411–26.

Johnson S. *Who Moved My Cheese?* New York: GP Putnam and Sons; 1998.

Kitson A. The multi-professional agenda and clinical effectiveness. In: Dieghan M, Hitch S, editors. *Clinical Effectiveness from Guidelines to Cost-Effective Practice.* Manchester: Health Service Management Unit; 1995.

Manangan LP, Pugliese G, Jackson M, *et al.* Infection control dogma: top 10 suspects. *Infect Control Hosp Epidemiol.* 2001; **22**: 243–7.

Medicines and Healthcare Products Regulatory Agency. *Community Equipment Loan Stores: guidance on decontamination.* London: MHRA; 2003.

National Audit Office. *The Management and Control of Hospital-Acquired Infection in NHS Acute Trusts in England.* London: The Stationery Office; 2000.

National Audit Office. *Improving Patient Care by Reducing the Risk of Hospital-Acquired Infection: a progress report.* London: The Stationery Office; 2004.

National Health Service Executive. *Controls Assurance Standard in Infection Control 1999 (rev 04).* London: The Stationery Office; 2001.

NHS Education for Scotland 2003. *Cleanliness Champions.* Available at: www.nes.scot.nhs.uk/hai/champions/ (accessed 25 Nov 2008).

Pellowe CM, Pratt RJ, Harper P, *et al.* Evidence-based guidelines for preventing healthcare-associated infections in primary and community care in England. *Br J Infect Control.* 2003; (Suppl.): S1–S118.

Pirwitz M, Manian F. Prevalence of use of infection control rituals and outdated practices: Education Committee survey results. *Am J Infect Control.* 1997; **25**: 28–33.

Pratt RJ, Pellowe C, Loveday HP, *et al.* The epic project: developing national evidence-based guidelines for preventing healthcare associated infections. Phase 1: guidelines for preventing hospital-acquired infections. *J Hosp Infect.* 2001; **47**(Suppl.): S3–S82.

Raven BH, Haley RW. Social influence and compliance of hospital nurses with infection control policies. In: Eiser R, editor. *Social Psychology and Behavioural Medicine.* Chichester: John Wiley; 1982.

Tew L, King D, Moore L, Meyers D. New horizons: developing the novice infection control nurse through work-based learning and the new professional core competencies. *Br J Infect Control.* 2002; **3**(4): 16–20.

The Commission for Health Improvement 2003. *Performance Ratings for NHS Trusts in England.* Available at: www.healthcarecommission.org.uk/homepage.cfm (accessed 25 Nov 2008).

Welsh Assembly 2004. *Healthcare Associated Infections: a strategy for hospitals in Wales.* Available at: www.wales.nhs.uk/sites3/documents/379/HAI-strategy.pdf (accessed 25 Nov 2008).

INTRODUCTION

Ben Waters is a senior lecturer in law at Canterbury Christ Church University with the Department of Law and Criminal Justice Studies. Ben and I first met through producing this book as I was particularly keen to have someone with Ben's expertise provide some input. In writing Chapter 3, Ben provides an interesting and perhaps enlightening perspective on the legal issues surrounding infection control, so you may want to reflect upon the legality of your own practice when reading through his chapter.

The legal issues relating to infection control

Ben Waters

INTRODUCTION

It's a Monday morning and the chief executive of a large NHS Trust has called a meeting of the hospital Trust Board for 2:00pm that day. The reason for calling the meeting is to announce that on the previous Friday the National Health Service Litigation Authority settled a claim brought by the estate of a patient who died a little more than two years ago as a result of a hospital-acquired infection whilst the patient was in one of the Trust's hospitals. Due to the advanced age of the patient the settlement was modest in relative terms, and upon the Trust's instructions their solicitors agreed to reach a compromise with the solicitors acting for the patient's executors. This means that many other settlements are likely to follow, as a result of similar cases, at great cost to the Trust and ultimately the tax payer. At the meeting the chief executive will provide estimated figures regarding the Trust's likely financial exposure if all known cases, either already indicated or anticipated where the Trust will be unable to successfully deny liability, will have to be settled. It will be an uncomfortable meeting for many reasons and there will be much soul searching and reflection. The Trust's culpability will mean that financial savings will have to be made from its NHS budget and this will undoubtedly lead to future healthcare cuts within the area administered by the Trust. The chief executive will ask a number of probing questions, many of which will focus on risk management. Questions, that is, which should have been asked more than two years ago before the 'stable door' was left wide open, resulting in the inevitable stampede.

This is, of course, a hypothetical scenario, but one which quite easily could be a reality. Increasing numbers of patients are dying from healthcare-acquired infections. Some of the more common of these are methicillin-resistant *Staphylococcus aureus* (MRSA), methicillin-sensitive *Staphylococcus aureus* (MSSA), vancomycin- or glycopeptide-resistant enterococci (VRE/GRE) and *Clostridium difficile* (*C. difficile*) (Weston 2008). These 'superbugs', as they have been termed by the media, have caused widespread infection in hospitals in the UK and abroad and have resulted in the deaths of thousands of patients in the UK alone (BBC News online, 22 February 2007). Weston (2008) points to the fact that many hospitals are no longer able to cope with the population they were originally built to serve and that higher bed occupancy rates, patient turnaround times and increased movement of patients between wards and departments places a huge demand on facilities and resources and inevitably impacts upon infection rates.

In this chapter, the core legal issues surrounding healthcare infection control will be outlined. This will include an examination of the circumstances that give rise to liability of the health and social care professionals, including residential and home care workers; where the law currently stands both in the context of tortious liability and in relation to the statutory framework governing hospitals as places of work; and the particular situations where criminal liability may arise due to recent changes in the law. The chapter will also highlight the inevitable costs that flow from negligence arising from both primary and secondary care provision, the risk management issues which have to be contemplated by every clinician and the effective strategies that must be implemented and maintained within every clinical healthcare environment to avoid the spectre of litigation. Reference will be made throughout this chapter to published statistics which, if relied upon as being accurate, are – in some cases – alarming.

THE GROWING THREAT OF HEALTHCARE-ACQUIRED INFECTION

Firstly let us examine the changing landscape concerning healthcare-acquired infection against which these legal issues should be considered. Herring (2006) takes the view that there are few things a patient awaiting treatment fears more: that the intervention, far from improving their condition, will make it worse. This may well be an accurate reflection of the fear a patient has of the surgical procedure, but what of the patient's fear of merely entering the hospital or a GP surgery as a patient or even receiving treatment at home in the social care environment? A more accurate and rational concern held not only by patients requiring surgical intervention in hospitals in the UK in the

21st century, but also by those coming into contact with anyone working in the clinical healthcare or social care environment, must be the fear of infection. The statistics speak for themselves. In England and Wales alone, between 1993 and 2006, 20 732 death certificates were completed with *Staphylococcus aureus* or MRSA being mentioned as the underlying cause of death, of which MRSA was responsible for just about 60% (Office of National Statistics). What is more alarming is that these figures are increasing steadily year by year. In 1993, 1025 death certificates were completed with *Staphylococcus aureus* and MRSA being mentioned as an underlying cause of death. In 2006, this figure was 3564, a rise of nearly 30% (Office of National Statistics).

The number of death certificates mentioning MRSA alone actually stabilised at 1652 in 2006, but this figure still far exceeds the number of pedestrians killed on our roads each year. In 2005, the number of pedestrian fatalities was 671 (Office of National Statistics). Based on these statistics a patient has a 60% higher chance of dying from MRSA infection than of being killed crossing the road to reach the hospital. These are the recent figures for one hospital-acquired infection and do not include others where perhaps a higher risk factor exists; for instance the recent rise in patient deaths related to *C. difficile* gives major cause for concern. In 2006 a staggering 6480 patients' death certificates either mentioned *C. difficile* or recorded the bacteria as being the underlying cause of death (Office of National Statistics). Therefore, the chances of contracting a hospital-acquired infection are significantly high.

In 2006, hospitals in the UK saw 55 681 cases of *C. difficile* in patients over 65 years old – a rise of 8% on the previous year's figures (Healthcare Commission 2007). Katherine Murphy, Director of Communications at the Patients' Association, quoted in the *British Medical Journal* by Michael Day, stated that:

> The [current] number of deaths from *C difficile* is equivalent to a packed jumbo jet crashing every month (Day 2007, p. 924).

She went on to ask when an NHS chief executive was actually going to lose his or her job over the failure to control the spread of hospital-acquired infection. She did not have to wait long for that question to be answered, because in October 2007 the Healthcare Commission published its long-awaited report into outbreaks of *C. difficile* at Maidstone & Tunbridge Wells NHS Trust in October and November 2005, when 150 known patients were affected. The report was damning: one conclusion was that the Trust had no effective system for surveillance of *C. difficile* and that its policy for responding to outbreaks was not fit for its intended purpose. As a consequence it missed the outbreak in 2005, which involved 150 patients, and the report concluded that *C. difficile* was definitely or probably the main cause of death for 90 patients (Healthcare Commission 2007). Shortly after the report was published, the Chief Executive of Maidstone & Tunbridge Wells NHS Trust resigned after the Commission considered that the Trust's Board should review its leadership (Healthcare Commission 2007) – a clear criticism of the chief executive herself. Claims will undoubtedly follow and the cost to the NHS is likely to be significant.

CIVIL LIABILITY FOR HEALTHCARE-ACQUIRED INFECTION
Breach of duty at common law

In order to prove negligence against a provider of health or social care services – be they a private hospital, nursing home, hospital NHS trust or a general practitioner (GP) – for a healthcare-acquired infection, it is necessary to firstly establish the existence of a common law duty of care. Secondly it is necessary to demonstrate that the duty of care has been breached, and thirdly, to show that a material loss has occurred. The claimant must prove, on the balance of probabilities, that the defendant's breach caused the damage (Khan, Robson and Swift 2002). In legal terms, this is commonly known as 'causation'.

The existence of a duty of care will be easy to establish. If healthcare treatment is provided for a patient, a legal relationship will arise between the provider and the patient. This may be a result of either primary care (the care provided at the first point of contact with the NHS), which is supervised by primary care Trusts, largely through general practitioners and other clinicians (especially dentists, nurses and pharmacists), or secondary care and NHS community care (hospital and community healthcare services) (Newdick 2005).

The breach of duty is somewhat more difficult to establish – whatever the context of the healthcare provision. The basis of the standard remains as that laid down in the case of *Bolam v Friern Hospital Management Committee* [1957] 2All ER 118. Based on the decision in that case, to prove that a clinician was negligent in the way that a patient was treated, the patient must be able to show that the treatment provided fell below the standard of practice accepted as proper by a responsible body of medical opinion skilled in that particular area of expertise. In the case of infection control, evidence would have to be obtained from expert witnesses, such as infection control nurses and microbiologists (Portsmouth 2007).

As well as proving 'negligent un-cleanliness' a patient will also need to show that the clinician failed to respond reasonably to the needs of the patient once the patient had tested positive for the infection. For example, according to Portsmouth (2007), failure to implement recognised risk reduction strategies once a case of *C. difficile* is recognised (e.g. isolating the patient in a single room, wearing gloves and aprons, using dedicated toileting facilities, reviewing antibiotic treatment or instigating environmental cleaning) could constitute practice falling below that considered to be the acceptable standard of care.

Healthcare professionals working in all clinical healthcare environments have a duty of care to ensure that hand decontamination is undertaken before and after direct patient contact. They also have a duty of care to ensure that reusable medical equipment is decontaminated appropriately between uses. This applies equally to complex pieces of equipment like endoscopes and surgical instruments, and to the less complex, such as commodes, urinals and bedpans – equipment that because of constant use can easily become contaminated with transient micro-organisms such as *C. difficile* and MRSA. Compliance with infection control practices and procedures is therefore essential if [a healthcare provider] is to avoid failing in the duty of care that has been established between the individual and the patient (Portsmouth 2007). Similarly, where nursing home patient care is concerned, such failings would also constitute an unacceptable level of practice.

The claimant must also prove causation; that is, on the balance of probabilities the defendant's breach caused the damage. The claimant will succeed if he or she can show that:

➤ The damage would not have occurred but for the defendant's negligence; or

➤ The defendant's negligence materially contributed to, or materially increased, the risk of injury (Khan, Robson and Swift 2002). This is sometimes known as the 'but for' test: but for the negligent act or omission, injury would not have occurred.

In a negligence case involving a patient claiming injury due to healthcare-acquired infection, a patient's legal action will fail unless it can be shown that it was more probable that the patient's injuries were caused by professional negligence in relation to the acquisition of the infection than by some other innocent cause (Montgomery 2003).

The question then arises: who will be liable if negligence can be proved? In the context of secondary care and NHS community and social care provision, since *Cassidy v Ministry of Health* [1951] 2 KB 343 the law imposes civil liability on the hospital, not the individual. In the case of *Cassidy* the court considered that a surgeon was an integral part of the organisation and so was an employee. Based on this decision, any employee considered to be an integral part of the organisation would be treated as an employee and as such an NHS Trust would, under the principle of vicarious liability, be liable for the employee's acts or omissions. GPs can be held individually liable for failing to reach the reasonable standards expected of *the average GP.*

Clinical governance

The level of care will also require a healthcare provider to ensure that it complies with relevant Guidelines and Codes of Practice issued within the NHS, laid down by the National Institute for Clinical Health and Excellence (NICE) or promoted by the Commission for Healthcare Improvement (McHale and Tingle 2002), which state 'best practice'. In other words, all clinicians must ensure that they maintain standards that are compliant with clinical governance. This includes clinical audit, evidence-based practice, clinical risk management, clinical effectiveness, clinical guidelines and professional self-regulation (Wilson cited in Hendrick 2004). A court will ordinarily regard failure to observe acceptable standards of clinical governance as evidence of breach of duty, unless non-compliance can be justified on the facts (Grubb and Laing 2004; *R v North Derbyshire HA, ex p Fisher* [1997] 8 Med LR 327). Newdick (2005) observes that before 2002, NICE had limited impact on health authorities because they were not bound to adopt its recommendations. Of course, such guidance had to be considered in the decision-making process, as indicted by the ruling in *ex p Fisher.* However, since 2002, NICE guidance has assumed the status of *Directions.* The impact of clinical governance on healthcare provision should therefore not be underestimated.

It is worth noting that a patient has the right to obtain their medical records pursuant to the Data Protection Act 1998, an Act that covers the processing of personal data. Under the provision of the Freedom of Information Act 2000, any patient could conceivably make a request to a health provider, be it a hospital, nursing home or GP surgery, for information in the records held by them. In the case of a hospital, such records could include the hospital's infection control policy. The provisions of this Act give citizens the right to access information held by public authorities and any person making a request for information to a public authority is entitled to be told in writing by the authority whether it holds the information, and if so, to have that information communicated to him or her (Stone 2004). An honest response to such a request may well reveal systemic shortcomings.

Breach of statutory duty

There are various statutory provisions that may impose liability on health and social care providers for the spread of infection. The Health and Safety at Work etc Act 1974 provides the statutory framework associated with occupational health and safety and imposes both civil and criminal liability on employers.

In the context of civil liability, imposed under *s.2* of the Act, is a general duty on employers to provide a safe system and place of work. *S.3* requires employers to ensure, as is reasonably practicable, that persons other than employees are not placed at risk by the way they conduct their work. Under *s.7* an employee has a general duty while at work to take reasonable care for the health and safety of himself and of other persons who may be affected by his acts or omissions at work.

A hospital or nursing home's liability can be viewed in terms of injury merely being an acquired infection rather than being due to a medical accident, by reference to the Control of Substances Hazardous to Health Regulations 1994 (COSHH). COSHH require employers to prevent or control exposure of employees and/or other people to hazardous substances, which include micro-organisms, biological, fungal and/or viral agents. Healthcare-acquired pathogens will fall into the category of micro-organisms and as such hospitals, nursing homes and GP surgeries must take steps to prevent exposure to infection from pathogens (Health and Safety Executive 2008).

It is arguable that the use of these particular regulations may well provide claimants with a far easier route to establishing liability rather than litigating at common law negligence (Bennett 2004). Litigating using COSHH, suggests Bennett (2004), has a number of significant advantages: there is no 'foreseeability' test; that is, the claimant does not have to prove that the organisation's failings were more than likely to cause injury or harm; the duties imposed upon organisations are strict and purposive; the burden of proving that the duties have been complied with is on the defendant organisation; and the causation test is the 'material increase in risk' test and not the previously mentioned 'but for' test applied at common law.

The *Management of Health and Safety at Work Regulations 1999*, which amended the earlier 1992 EC directive to bring it into line with the European health and safety framework, requires employers to undertake risk assessments and take preventative and protective measures (Health and Safety Executive 2008). Therefore, failure by health or social care providers to demonstrate a strict regime of risk assessment in relation to the control and spread of pathogens will give rise to a breach.

Part 2 of the Health Act (2006) amends the Health and Social Care (Community Health and Standards) Act (2003), creating a new *s.47A*, which allows the Secretary of State for Health to issue a Code of Practice to all healthcare Trusts relating to healthcare-acquried infections. This can impose important obligations on Trusts to ensure that they safeguard individuals from the risk of being exposed to healthcare-acquired infections. It gives the Commission for Healthcare Audit and Inspection (CHAI) the power to serve an improvement notice on the hospital in the event of failure to observe the code (Department of Health 2006).

CRIMINAL LIABILITY FOR HEALTHCARE-ACQUIRED INFECTION

At common law criminal liability for negligence is effectively limited to prosecutions for manslaughter, where there has been gross or extreme negligence (Mason and McCall Smith 2006). The standard of proof for such cases has been confirmed in *R v Bateman* ([1925] All ER Rep 45 at 48) by Lord Hewart LCJ, who stated that:

> In order to establish criminal liability, the facts must be such that [...] the negligence of the accused went beyond a mere matter of compensation between subjects and showed such disregard for the life and the safety of others as to amount to a crime against the State and conduct deserving of punishment.

The law is aimed at individuals and if a health and safety offence is committed with the consent or connivance of, or is attributable to any neglect on the part of any director, manager, secretary or other similar officer of the organisation, then that person (as well as the organisation) can be prosecuted under *s.37* of the Health and Safety at Work etc Act 1974. This provision will apply equally to hospitals, nursing homes and GP surgeries.

Apart from the very limited circumstances set out in the legislation described so far, up until 6 April 2008 a healthcare organisation could not be criminally liable for deaths of patients whilst in their care, but since this date the Corporate Manslaughter and Corporate Homicide Act 2007 has been in force and extends the scope of criminal liability to organisations including Department of Health NHS Trusts and other corporate entities providing health or social care services. The Act introduces a new offence across the UK for prosecuting companies and other organisations where there has been a gross failing, throughout the organisation, in the management of health and safety with fatal consequences. This will mean that a trust or nursing home could be held criminally liable for the deaths of thousands of patients who die of healthcare-acquired infection if it can be shown that the organisation acted in such a way that its activities were managed or organised to cause a person's death, and that these activities amounted to a gross breach of a relevant duty of care owed by the organisation to the deceased.

THE IMPACT UPON HEALTHCARE AND THE COMMUNITY

The cost of healthcare providers and those in the social care sector failing to adequately manage infection control not only impacts in loss of life, but also inevitably in financial terms as well. This, in turn, has a knock-on effect to the provision of effective healthcare services to the community.

During 2006–07, clinical negligence claims cost the government over £613 million in payments made by the NHS Litigation Authority (NHSLA) for damages and legal costs (NHSLA Annual Report 2007). In January 2008, the NHSLA announced that it had made a compensation payment of £5 million to the actress Lesley Ash, which set a new record for compensation in a case of hospital-acquired infection, adding that the size reflected her prospective future loss of earnings (*The Times* 17 January 2008). Many more such payments could have a profound effect on healthcare provision.

Since 1990, NHS Trusts have been responsible for meeting the costs involved in hospital litigation; they are not permitted to take out insurance to cover malpractice costs (Montgomery 2003). Although the Clinical Negligence Scheme for Trusts was established in 1995 in order to create a pooling arrangement to meet claims brought by NHS patients, premiums are based on the type of Trust, the specialities offered and the scale of operations. Also, risk management procedures have to be complied with (Brazier and Cave 2007). Where a claim is made by an NHS patient, money to compensate the injured patient – and money to defend the claims brought in respect of the alleged negligence – must come out of NHS funds, which might otherwise have been used to employ an extra surgeon, pay for a new neo-natal unit or support a programme of preventative medicine (Merry and McCall Smith 2001). Therefore, the cost of meeting claims brought by patients undoubtedly has a detrimental effect on the Trust's ability to fund its frontline healthcare services. Cost cutting is the inevitable consequence of negligence.

It could be argued that it is irresponsible for an NHS Trust or a social care provider to fail in its provision of a service to the extent that it falls short of the standards required to prevent the spread of infection. Risk management is vital in order to prevent the spread of infection – a view supported by Cranfield (2006) who, in the context of the delivery of healthcare, defines risk management as the identification, analysis and control of potential adverse outcomes that threaten the proper delivery of healthcare to patients. An effective risk management programme will therefore be based on identity, measurement, control and monitoring. If NHS hospitals fail to have such risk management strategies in place to deal with infection control, they are failing not only themselves but also their patients, and are exposing themselves to the kind of legislative responses outlined in this chapter.

CONCLUSION

Whilst the bar is undoubtedly set high for a patient to succeed in a negligence action against a healthcare or social care provider, whether employed or acting privately, for an acquired infection at common law, the tightening of regulation as a result of legislative developments, clinical governance and the threat of potential criminal liability sends a clear message to hospitals. Now healthcare providers and those providing social care are required to be ever more vigilant in their risk management procedures if claims of healthcare-acquired infection and the inevitable adverse consequences are to be avoided.

REFERENCES

BBC News Online. Hospital bug deaths on the rise. 22 Feb 2007. Available at: http://news.bbc.co.uk/1/hi/health/6385323.stm (accessed 25 Nov 2008).

Bennett D. Litigating hospital-acquired MRSA as a disease. *JPIL.* 2004; 3: 197–208.

Bolam v Friern Hospital Management Committee [1957] 2A11 Er118.

Brazier M, Cave E. *Medicine, Patients and the Law.* 4th ed. New York: Penguin Books; 2007.

Cassidy v Ministry of Health [1951] 2 KB343.

Control of Substances Hazardous to Health Regulations (COSHH) 1974. Available at: www.opsi.gov.uk/si/si2002/20022677.htm (accessed 25 Nov 2008).

Corporate Manslaughter and Corporate Homicide Act 2007. Available at: www.hse.gov.uk (accessed 25 Nov 2008).

Cranfield F. Risk management in general practice. In: Palmer R, Wetherill D, editors. *Medicine for Lawyers.* London: The Royal Society for Medicine Press Limited; 2005.

Data Protection Act 1998. Available at: www.opsi.gov.uk/Acts/Acts1998/ukpga_19980029_en_1 (accessed 25 Nov 2008).

Day M. *C difficile* infections rise – but MRSA rates drop. *BMJ.* 2007; 334(7600): 924.

Department of Health. *Health Act 2006: code of practice for the prevention and control of healthcare-associated infections.* London: HMSO; 2006.

Freedom of Information Act 2000. Available at: www.opsi.gov.uk/Acts/acts2000/ukpga_20000036_en_1 (accessed 25 Nov 2008).

Grubb A, Laing J. *Principles of Medical Law.* 2nd ed. Oxford: Oxford University Press; 2004.

Health Act 2006. Available at www.opsi.gov.uk/acts/acts2006/pdf/ukpga_20060028_en.pdf (accessed 25 Nov 2008).

Health and Safety at Work etc Act 1974. Available at www.hse.gov.uk/legislation/hswa.pdf (accessed 25 Nov 2008).

Health and Safety Executive. Available at www.hse.gov.uk (accessed 25 Nov 2008).

Health and Social Care (Community Health and Standards) Act 2003. Available at: www.opsi.gov.uk/acts/acts2003/ukpga_20030043_en_1 (accessed 25 Nov 2008).

Healthcare Commission. *Investigation into Outbreaks of Clostridium difficile at Maidstone & Tunbridge Wells NHS Trust.* 2007. Available at www.healthcarecommission.org.uk (accessed 25 Nov 2008).

Herring J. *Medical Law and Ethics.* 2nd ed. Oxford: Oxford University Press; 2006.

Khan M, Robson M, Swift, K. *Clinical Negligence.* 2nd ed. London: Cavendish; 2002.

McHale J, Tingle J. *Law and Nursing.* 2nd ed. Oxford: Butterworth/Heinemann; 2002.

Management of Health and Safety at Work Regulations 1999. Available at www.hse.gov.uk (accessed 25 Nov 2008).

Mason J, McCall Smith R. *Medical Law and Ethics.* 7th ed. London: Butterworths; 2006.

Merry A, McCall Smith A. *Errors, Medicine and the Law.* London: Cambridge University Press; 2001.

Montgomery J. *Healthcare Law.* 2nd ed. Oxford: Oxford University Press; 2003.

National Health Service Litigation Authority Annual Report 2007. Available at www.nhsla.com (accessed 25 Nov 2008).

Newdick C. *Who Should We Treat?: rights, rationing, and resources in the NHS.* Oxford: Oxford University Press; 2005.

Office of National Statistics. *Clostridium difficile:* number of deaths increase in 2007. 28 August 2008. Available at: www.statistics.gov.uk/cci/nugget.asp?id=1735.

Office of National Statistics. MRSA: deaths decrease in 2007. 28 August 2008. Available at: www.statistics.gov.uk/CCI/nugget.asp?ID=1067.

Office of National Statistics. Road casualties: pedestrian deaths at 40 year low. 31 July 2006. Available at: www.statistics.gov.uk/cci/nugget.asp?id=1208.

Portsmouth J. Infection control and the law: legal and ethical obligations. *Br J Infect Control.* 2007; 8(2): 14–19.

R v Bateman [1925] A11 ER Rep 45 at 48.

R v North Derbyshire HA, ex p Fisher [1997] 8 Med LR 327.

Sanderson D, Gibb E. Leslie Ash gets £5m pound payout from hospital where she caught infection. *The Times.* 17 Jan 2008. Available at www.timesonline.co.uk/tol/life_and_style/health/article3201003.ece (accessed 25 Nov 2008).

Stone R. *Textbook on Civil Liberties and Human Rights.* 5th ed. Oxford: Oxford University Press; 2004.

Weston D. *Infection Prevention and Control: theory and practice for healthcare professionals.* Chichester: John Wiley; 2008.

Wilson J. Clinical governance: the legal perspective. In: Tingle, J and Cribb A, editors. *Nursing Law and Ethics.* 2nd ed. Oxford: Blackwell Science; 2002. Referred to by Hendrick J in Law and Ethics: foundations in nursing and healthcare. Cheltenham: Nelson Thornes; 2004.

CHAPTER 4

Biomedical versus biopsychosocial perspectives

Before reading this chapter take some time to think about how you would define the terms 'biomedical' and 'biopsychosocial' and their relevance to infection control practice.

You might want to write your thoughts and feelings down so you can refer back to them as you work through this chapter.

This chapter will reflect upon the principles underlying the biomedical and biopsychosocial approaches to health (Ogden 2007) and their application to infection control practice. I will argue that the application of a biomedical approach (*see* List 4.1) promotes unsafe infection control practice and that those health and social care professionals who adopt a biomedical approach are responsible for placing themselves and others at risk. Further, in adopting a biomedical approach, health and social care professionals are responsible for increased rates of cross infection; increased physical, psychological and social suffering for patients and clients; increased economic burdens; and higher mortality rates.

LIST 4.1 RELATING THE BIOMEDICAL MODEL TO INFECTION CONTROL

This model (Elliott and BVS Training 2005) assumes that:

1   The concepts of health and illness are seen to exist separately.
    Infection control example: Healthcare-acquired infection and the interventions made by health and social care professionals are seen as existing in isolation; they are not perceived as impacting upon each other.

2   Disease or infection is external to the body and is not the result of an individual's behaviour.
    Infection control example: The behaviour of health and social care professionals has no impact upon the risk of cross infection.

3   Individuals should have no control over or involvement with what happens to them regarding their health and wellbeing.
    Infection control example: Patients and clients have no right to question or challenge health and social care professionals even though the patient or client may have contracted a healthcare-acquired infection through the health or social care professional's negligence as a result of their poor and inadequate adoption of standard precautions.

4   Individuals have no responsibility to ensure the maintenance of their own or others' health and wellbeing.
    Infection control example: Despite failing to adopt standard precautions, health and social care professionals are not responsible for the consequences of such a failure.

5   Although it is acknowledged they exist, the mind and body are perceived as being separate with neither having consequences for the other.
    Infection control example: A health and social care professional who is experiencing stress will demonstrate a greater propensity towards becoming cognitively economic (*see* Explanation box 4.1) and unrealistically optimistic (*see* Explanation box 4.2) in their perception of the importance of standard precautions. Despite this, there will be no impact upon their behaviour; therefore, a failure to carry out standard precautions according to a bio-medical perspective is not a consequence of the way a health or social care professional thinks but simply a physical action.

6   Psychosocial factors have no part to play and healthcare intervention should centre around the physical aspects in isolation.
    Infection control example: Healthcare-acquired infection has nothing to do with how health and social care professionals think or the social context within which they are practising. Cross infection is simply a consequence of the physical factors, such as the cleanliness of equipment, the environment or staff uniforms/work clothing.

7   Health and social care professionals are knowledgeable experts who always
    know best.
    Infection control example: Attitudes such as 'I am safe', 'I am competent', 'I
    know what I am doing' or 'I am an expert' are all indicative of dissonance-
    based thinking (*see* Explanation box 4.3) and a cognitively economic
    perspective (*see* Explanation box 4.1) towards their ability to carry out
    consistent safe infection control practice. However, terms such as 'safe',
    'competent' and 'expert' are all spurious in nature and are reflective of an
    egocentric and conceited self-perception, which serves to precipitate unsafe
    infection-control behaviour.

8   Patients and clients cease to have their own identity. Rather they become
    stereotyped or labelled by health and social care professionals.
    Infection control example: Patients and clients who contract a healthcare-
    acquired infection may be seen as the health problem they present with in
    isolation, as opposed to a person in their own right. For example, an indi-
    vidual with methicillin-resistant *Staphylococcus aureus* (MRSA) loses the
    right to be seen as a person and becomes an entity. This entity principle has
    particular relevance when a patient or client having contracted a healthcare-
    acquired infection is placed in a side room, becomes perceived as dirty and
    are then forgotten – out of sight and out of mind!

9   It is acceptable to ridicule a patient or client when they fail to conform to
    the assumptions, expectations or requirements of health and social care
    professionals.
    Infection control example: Patients and clients who experience a healthcare-
    acquired infection become stigmatised by health and social care professionals
    who may originally have been responsible for them contracting an infection
    in the first place. As a result of such they are perceived as failing to conform
    with the expectations of those health and social care professionals.

NB: The above should not be seen as being mutually exclusive, but rather as
providing a perspective.

EXPLANATION BOX 4.1 COGNITIVE ECONOMY
(ROTH AND FRISBY 1992)

Cognitive economy is where an individual has become context-specific or
tunnel-visioned in their perception of what is occurring around them and will
fail to take into account the wider implications of their behaviour. For example,
instead of being patient-centred, the individual will become task-orientated

towards achieving a set of goals that will meet their own needs at the expense of everything else and the needs of others.

Example: In the case of standard precautions, the individual will be context-specific towards achieving their allocated work load and as a result of this may:

- fail to change their gloves between interventions;
- fail to undertake or to fully follow the hand hygiene process;
- fail to ensure that they have removed all the equipment they used following completion of a procedure.

EXPLANATION BOX 4.2 UNREALISTIC OPTIMISM (OGDEN 2007)

Unrealistic optimism is where a health or social care professional becomes unrealistically optimistic regarding risky situations they place themselves and others in as a result of behaviour that constitutes unsafe infection control practice in the form of failing to undertake standard precautions (*see* Table 4.1) or through failing to follow the hand hygiene process (*see* List 4.4).

Unrealistic optimism can be facilitated through lack of personal experience. For example, a health or social care professional who has no prior experience of a patient's or client's health being directly influenced by their failure to adopt appropriate standard precautions will likely believe two things (Elliott 2003a):

1 There is no risk, or the risk of cross infecting others is so insignificant that it simply does not matter.
2 Even if there is a risk it will not happen to them. That is, even if the individual involved in healthcare does cross infect others they will rationalise that is was not their fault (*see* Explanation box 4.3) or they will not be found out and held responsible and therefore, who cares?

EXPLANATION BOX 4.3 COGNITIVE DISSONANCE

The concept of cognitive dissonance was originally identified by Festinger (1962), where he proposed that at a psychological level the individual will strive to make consistent two or more things that would not naturally be so. In simple terms, dissonance effects are when an individual generates excuses to justify their previous behaviour or behaviour they wish or intend to carry out; for example, hand hygiene. The individual understands the importance of hand hygiene in reducing cross infection, yet fails to adequately follow the hand hygiene process. Thus the individual experiences conflict between knowing what they should do and what they actually do or want to do.

Such conflict would be manifested as stress in the individual. In an attempt to reduce such stress the individual will generate an excuse or reason for failing to follow the hand hygiene process. Such an excuse may be blamed on time, work load or a belief that meeting others' needs must take priority.

In contrast to the biomedical approach (*see* List 4.1) the adoption of a bio-psychosocial approach (*see* List 4.2) by health and social care professionals can improve the quality of infection control practice, help to reduce rates of cross infection and levels of non-adherence to standard precautions, reduce levels of physical; psychological and social suffering for patients and clients and have a positive impact upon economic, resourcing and mortality rates. For example, adopting a biomedical approach will cause health and social care professionals to dehumanise the patient or client by taking their individuality away from them. Further, adopting a biomedical approach will focus the health and social care professional's attention upon the physical needs of an individual. However, the adoption of a biopsychosocial approach will promote individuality through recognising that the patient or client is an integral part of the health and social care team. Further, adopting a biopsychosocial approach will focus attention towards the importance of meeting the patient or client's physical, psychological and social needs.

LIST 4.2 RELATING THE BIOPSYCHOSOCIAL MODEL TO INFECTION CONTROL

This model (Elliott and BVS Training 2005) assumes that:

1 The concepts of health and illness are perceived as coexisting on a continuum.

    Infection control example: The contracting of a healthcare-acquired infection will impact upon different individuals' life spans and ability to carry out their activities of daily living (Roper, Logan and Tierney 2000).

2 Infection can be internal or external to the body and may be the result of an individual's health behaviour.

    Infection control example: An internal cause of infection may be the result of a patient or client's behaviour. An external cause of infection may be the result of the behaviour of health and social care professionals. Both of these may lead to the contracting of a healthcare-acquired infection.

3 Patients and clients should be offered the opportunity to be actively involved

in the decision-making process with regard to their health and wellbeing.
Infection control example: Patients and clients should be actively encouraged
to challenge and question the judgements and decisions of health and social
care professionals with regard to the degree to which they apply the principles of safe infection control practice. If a health and social care professional
fails to facilitate such, they may well find themselves in contravention of a
patient or client's human rights.

4 Individuals should accept responsibility for their own health behaviour.
Infection control example: Health and social care professionals must accept
responsibility for their health behaviour from two standpoints:
- accepting responsibility for the quality and standard of their infection
  control practice;
- accepting responsibility for their own health and wellbeing. For
  example, if they are unwell and aware that they may be infectious then
  they should act in an appropriate professional manner.

5 The physical, psychological and social aspects that make up an individual
coexist, with each having the potential to impact upon the other.
Infection control example: Failing to adopt standard precautions will have
physical, psychological and social consequences for health and social care
professionals, patients and clients, and for society as a whole.

6 Psychosocial factors carry equal importance to physical factors with regard
to healthcare intervention.
Infection control example: Where the adoption of standard precautions are
concerned health and social care professionals must recognise that they
will have physical, psychological and social implications for patients and
clients.

7 Patients and clients may have a greater knowledge of their health problem
than the health and social care professionals.
Infection control example: Health and social care professionals should work
in partnership with patients and clients with the aim of ensuring that standard precautions occur on a consistent basis.

8 Patients and clients should be empowered towards retaining their own
identity whilst receiving healthcare intervention.
Infection control example: Facilitating an individual towards retaining their
own identity as opposed to conditioning/categorising them into the patient
role will empower them towards questioning and challenging poor infection
control practice when it occurs.

9 If health and social care professionals fail to recognise the necessity of
a biopsychosocial approach, this can cause life-span consequences for
patients and clients.

Infection control example: The appropriate adoption of standard precautions by health and social care professionals has important implications regarding the future physical, psychological and social aspects of an individual's life span.

Historically the biomedical model has approached health and social care from a physical or physiological perspective whilst failing to account for the psychosocial aspects. This is consistent with Point 6 of List 4.1. In essence, the basic premise of the biomedical perspective is that the patient or client should be passive and accept without question the health and social care professionals' judgements, decisions and practices, believing them to know what they are doing. This is consistent with Points 3 and 7 of List 4.1. Within infection control, a biomedical approach continues to be adopted and this is clearly evident from the chain of infection (*see* List 4.3). Why? Because the chain of infection is physically/physiologically orientated. Nowhere within the content of the chain of infection is there any indication of psychological or social factors that serve to promote cross infection.

LIST 4.3 THE CHAIN OF INFECTION

The chain of infection is made up of various components:
1 Infectious agent: e.g. health and social care professionals.
2 Reservoirs: e.g. objects, enclosed spaces where close proximity exists between people.
3 Portals of entry to the person: e.g. wounds, inhalation, physical contact, ingestion.
4 Portals of exit from the person: e.g. coughing, sneezing, elimination, wounds.
5 Susceptible host: e.g. autoimmune, post-operative.
6 Mode of transmission: e.g. disregard of standard precautions.

NB: The above should not be seen as being mutually exclusive but as examples.

However, there may be many who would disagree with this by arguing that the chain of infection has made a contribution to reducing cross infection. Yet, there is no empirical evidence to show that the chain of infection has made any contribution to reducing cross infection or reducing the rates of healthcare-acquired infections. Despite this, the chain of infection continues to be widely promoted as a model of value. In reality it is an outdated and outmoded model that contributes nothing towards enhancing safe infection control practice.

Take some time to read through List 4.1.

Compare each of the points with your current infection control practice. Write down any similarities/differences that you find.

How biomedical is your infection control practice?

Having undertaken the above, reflect upon how person-centred your infection control practice is. Have there been instances when you have placed those around you at risk of cross infection as a result of your actions or omissions?

The argument that adopting a biomedical approach can also be person-centred is flawed (Elliott 2003b) and dissonance-based (Explanation box 4.3).Very little infection control practice is person-centred and remains task-orientated. Many health and social care professionals believe they are adopting a person-centred approach whilst adopting a biomedical approach.

The excuses and beliefs referred to in Explanation box 4.3 are irrational. For example, a practitioner fails to wash their hands between completing the dressing of an infected wound and the handling of food. When challenged, the abrasive response was, 'I am too busy meeting my patient's needs to worry about washing my hands'! (Elliott 2003a).

A second example of an irrational and dangerous belief about someone's practice being person-centred occurred a number of years ago whilst I was carrying out research within a regional South Wales hospital (Elliott 1996). In answer to one of the questions, a practitioner responded, 'I am too busy preparing for a theatre list to worry about washing my hands'!

Such comments are concerning and undoubtedly dissonance-based (*see* Explanation box 4.3). Further, such irrational beliefs are consistent with a biomedical approach where patients and clients are expected to accept the practitioner as a knowledgeable expert (*see* List 4.1, Points 3 and 7). However, such beliefs clearly indicate that far from being knowledgeable experts, many health and social care professionals are consistently dangerous in their infection control behaviour and increase the risk of cross infection to themselves and others within their working environment. For example, within operating departments, practitioners were found to be going outside between surgical cases in their theatre attire for a cigarette and then returning for the next case

(O'Dowd 2006). Apart from the legal, ethical, moral or human rights issues resulting from such behaviour, there can be no doubt that such actions constitute functioning at a biomedical level (*see* List 4.1, Point 2).

In linking the concepts inherent within a biomedical approach (*see* List 4.1) to the principles of standard precautions (*see* Table 4.1), it is clear that the application of this model results in unsafe practice and will serve to increase healthcare-acquired infections.

TABLE 4.1 Linking biomedical approaches to the application of standard precautions

Approaches underlying the biomedical model	Standard precautions	Identifying links between approaches and precautions
Facilitates a context-specific approach to care resulting in cognitively economic thinking	Management of sharps	Failing to perceive potential/actual dangers inherent in the handling of sharps
	Hand hygiene	Failing to recognise that adopting appropriate hand hygiene is an essential component of meeting an individual's needs
	Use of gloves	Believing that gloves will guarantee 100% protection
	Hygienic practice	Believing that completing a set work load will automatically indicate that such practice has been of an acceptable standard
Promotes paternalistic and task-orientated practice	Use of gloves	Failing to change gloves between tasks or failure to undertake hand hygiene between glove changes
	Hand hygiene	Health and social care professionals become defensive and present negative attitudes when asked by patients or clients if they have washed their hands
	Hygienic practice	Failing to recognise the difference between what constitutes socially clean, antiseptic and surgical practice
		Failing to undertake appropriate hygienic practice
	Disposal of waste	Believing that it is acceptable to ask or expect another to clear up the waste they have generated

(continued)

Approaches underlying the biomedical model	Standard precautions	Identifying links between approaches and precautions
Promotes the application of an external health locus of control	Hand hygiene	Excluding or refusing the patient's or client's right to question and challenge
	Use of gloves	Failing to explain to the patient or client why gloves are being worn
		Failing to explain to the patient or client that following their discharge it may be necessary for them to wear gloves when self-caring
	Personal clothing and protective clothing	Failing to recognise the purpose of protective clothing
		Failing to recognise the need to remove work and protective clothing prior to leaving their working environment
		Failing to recognise the risks to the general population when wearing work or protective clothing outside of the working environment (O'Dowd 2006)
	Handling of sharps	Failing to ensure that sharps are safely removed from the environment in which they were used
Facilitates inappropriate communication	Management of sharps and hygienic practice	Making the assumption that it is acceptable practice to expect one individual to clear away another's rubbish or sharps
	Disposal of waste	Failing to utilise the correctly coloured bag or container, or the correct waste
		Incorrect positioning of coloured bags or sharps containers within inappropriate environments
Facilitates the individual in becoming unrealistically optimistic whilst promoting dissonance effects	Personal clothing and protective clothing	Believing that a plastic apron will prevent contamination of a uniform or clothing
		Believing that the wearing of a plastic apron will prevent cross infection
	Hand hygiene	Believing that your practice is safe when it is clearly not

Approaches underlying the biomedical model	Standard precautions	Identifying links between approaches and precautions
		Failing to recognise that what we do when observed by others (role modelling) can be a powerful way of promoting the continuance of unsafe practice
	Use of gloves	Believing that the wearing of gloves will give 100% protection
		Believing that hand hygiene is not necessary when gloves are worn or that hand rub gels/solutions are an absolute substitute for formal hand hygiene
	Hygienic practice	Failing to recognise that clothing and equipment can increase the risk of cross infection
		Failing to recognise that because one's role does not involve physically touching a patient or client standard precautions are still necessary
Promotes stereotyping and labelling by those involved in the provision of healthcare	Use of gloves	Believing that the wearing of gloves is necessary for all aspects of clinical practice
	Hygienic practice	The belief that meeting someone's needs does not necessarily include the adoption of hand hygiene
		Believing that healthcare-acquired infection is an inevitable consequence of healthcare intervention, so why bother?
		Failing to recognise that infection control is everyone's responsibility
		Holding the belief that domestic hygiene is the sole responsibility of specifically employed cleaners
		Adopting the attitude that antiseptic practice is not essential when performing an invasive procedure – during cannulation or venepuncture

(continued)

Approaches underlying the biomedical model	Standard precautions	Identifying links between approaches and precautions
	Personal clothing and protective clothing	Holding the belief that a patient's or client's clothing will constitute a cross-infection risk whilst failing to recognise that work and protective clothing will constitute the exact same risk
	Disposal of waste	Failing to recognise that using the hands to open a waste container as opposed to lifting the container's lid using the foot pedal will not constitute a cross-infection risk
Facilitates a loss of individuality among recipients of healthcare resulting from the expectations and requirements imposed by those involved in the provision of healthcare	Hygienic practice	Failing to recognise and acknowledge that the patient or client will have a role to play in reducing the risk of cross infection

NB: The information in Table 4.1 should not be seen as being mutually exclusive, but rather as providing a perspective.

In contrast, a biopsychosocial approach when applied to standard precautions (Table 4.2) will increase understanding that unsafe practice has life span-related physical, psychological and social consequences for those contracting a healthcare-acquired infection. In consideration of this, health and social care professionals need to reflect far more on the consequences of failing to adopt a biopsychosocial approach.

TABLE 4.2 Linking biopsychosocial approaches to the application of standard precautions

Approaches underlying the biopsychosocial model	Standard precautions	Identifying links between approaches and precautions
Facilitates and promotes a multidirectional perspective	Management of sharps	Recognises the dangers and consequences to themselves and others of failing to correctly handle sharp objects
	Hand hygiene	Recognises that adopting hand hygiene is simply not enough. Understands that appropriate hand hygiene constitutes following all aspects of the hand hygiene process (*see* List 4.4)

Approaches underlying the biopsychosocial model	Standard precautions	Identifying links between approaches and precautions
	Use of gloves	Recognises that gloves are not an absolute barrier to contamination and that hand hygiene should be adopted both before applying and after removing gloves
	Disposal of waste	Recognises that all waste is a potential source of contamination and that appropriate disposal is essential
	Personal clothing and protective clothing	Recognises the importance of changing work clothing on a daily basis
		Recognises the questionability of wearing worn/soiled work clothing home from a place of work
		Recognises the dangers and risks of cross infection in wearing worn/soiled work clothing within social settings other than their normal working environment; e.g. leaving work and going into food retailers/shops
		Recognises the importance of protective clothing within the work place; e.g. disposable aprons and gloves
		Recognises the importance of changing protective clothing frequently irrespective of whether or not it is visibly soiled
	Hygienic practice	Recognises the importance of maintaining appropriate standards of personal hygiene
Promotes an internal locus of control and person-centred approach	Use of gloves	Health and social care professionals understand the importance of explaining to patients and clients why gloves are necessary for their protection
	Hand hygiene	Seeks to encourage patients and clients to question the hand hygiene practice of health and social care professionals
	Management of sharps and disposal of waste	Ensuring that the methods used for the disposal of sharps and waste is consistent with their employer's policies and Health and Safety Law (Taylor 2002)

(continued)

Approaches underlying the biopsychosocial model	Standard precautions	Identifying links between approaches and precautions
	Personal clothing and protective clothing	Raising awareness that the colour or type of work attire worn should not be taken as an indicator of knowledge, skill or experience. Not all those wearing white coats are doctors
Facilitates appropriate communication	Management of sharps, disposal of waste and hygienic practice	Ensuring that relevant communication occurs at an interprofessional level. Failing to inform would be a breach of human rights (Wilkinson and Caulfield 2001)
		Understanding that infection control is everyone's responsibility
Facilitates the individual in becoming more self-aware	Hand hygiene	Being familiar with the hand hygiene process (*see* List 4.4)
	Management of sharps and disposal of waste	Being observant to the non-adherent behaviour of colleagues and bringing such to their attention
	Use of gloves	Being aware that gloves are not an absolute barrier to cross infection
	Personal clothing and protective clothing	Being aware that not all contamination will be visible to the naked eye. Just because an item of clothing looks clean does not mean that it is
Can serve to reduce stereotyping and labelling by those involved in the provision of healthcare	Personal appearance	It would be inappropriate to stereotype or label a patient, client or colleague as unclean simply because they have not, e.g. shaved or are not neatly presented
	Hand hygiene	It would be inappropriate to stereotype or label a patient or client as disruptive or argumentative simply because they challenge or question your adoption of hand hygiene
	Handling of sharps and disposal of waste	It would be both inappropriate and unsafe to adopt the stereotypical attitude that contaminated waste and sharps are all going for incineration and therefore it is acceptable to dispose of both in the same bag or container

Approaches underlying the biopsychosocial model	Standard precautions	Identifying links between approaches and precautions
Promotes appropriate infection-control behaviour	Hand hygiene	A recognition by health and social care professionals that for the general population they will be role models with regard to their infection-control standards. What a patient or client observes you do will be interpreted as the correct way of doing things. Why? Because you are the health and social care professional and should know what you are doing

NB: The above should not be seen as being mutually exclusive but rather as providing a perspective.

However, it is not just patients or clients who can suffer the consequences of healthcare-acquired infections. Health and social care professionals need to be much more alert to the fact that they are not immune to cross infection as a result of their non-adherence to standard precautions. Such non-adherence will impact upon not only their health and wellbeing, but also the health and wellbeing of their family and friends. Yet many health and social care professionals negate the risk of contracting a healthcare-acquired infection by functioning at the level of 'It will not happen to me' (Elliott 2003a). This is a further example of a dissonance-based irrational belief (*see* Explanation box 4.3), which is again consistent with a biomedical approach.

In adopting a biomedical approach, failing to adhere to standard precautions and negating the risks of contracting a healthcare-acquired infection to such irrational beliefs, one can only surmise that most health and social care professionals care little about the patients' and clients' health and wellbeing, and perhaps more surprisingly the health and wellbeing of their own family and friends. However, when required to do so, every health and social care professional is likely to vehemently profess to care about the importance of not cross infecting others. Yet if they care so much, why is it that many of those working within the healthcare sector regularly attend their place of work with infectious illnesses? In reflecting upon such failings, it would seem that they emanate out of a complete disinterest in the ethics of knowingly cross infecting and causing harm to others (Seedhouse 1998).

Within the context of human rights (Wilkinson and Caulfield 2001), such knowledgeable actions (going to work knowing you are infectious) or omissions (failing to adopt standard precautions) have clear implications under Articles 2 and 3 of the Human Rights Act (1998) which came into force by Royal Assent in 2000 and gave individuals the right to make claims under the European Convention of Human Rights. Under Article 2 of the Act, each individual has a right to life and that their life should be protected when, for example, they are under the care of those involved in the provision of health-care. However, if an individual fails, through an act of omission (Sampson 2006), to adopt appropriate standard precautions or they knowingly place themselves in a position where they may or actually do pass on an infection or illness that they themselves are suffering from to a recipient of healthcare, then it might be argued by a recipient of healthcare that their right to life had potentially been infringed as a result of the individual involved in the provision of healthcare failing to take appropriate preventative measures.

Under Article 3, an individual has the right not to be subjected to torture where torture might be defined as the deliberate act of causing either physical, psychological or social pain or all three through an act of omission (Sampson 2006). Within the context of infection control, such an act might be a knowledgeable failure on the part of an individual involved in the provision of healthcare to adopt appropriate hand hygiene (*see* List 4.4) where such a failure leads to a recipient of healthcare contracting a healthcare-acquired infection. In such a case, the recipient of healthcare would undoubtedly be likely to experience physical, psychological and social pain through, for example, an enforced extended stay within a healthcare establishment, and anxiety, emotional distress and social isolation within a single room environment. The pain suffered by the patient or client as a result of the individual involved in healthcare failing to adopt the preventative measure of appropriate hand hygiene might be defined as a form of degrading treatment and thus, a form of torture.

Both of the above examples must be seen as falling within the context of a biomedical approach (*see* List 4.1, Points 4 and 6).

LIST 4.4 HAND HYGIENE PROCESS (ELLIOTT 2003a)

Stage 1 – It is vital that you recognise the need to undertake hand hygiene. This is probably the most important stage within the process because if you fail to recognise situations where you need to adopt formal hand hygiene as opposed to using hand cleansing rubs/gels, then the remainder of the process will at worst not occur or at best occur intermittently. Either way the risk of cross infection will be increased.

Stage 2 – It is important that you thoroughly wet all areas to be washed with running water. Failure do this may lead to you experiencing skin problems because some cleansing agents can cause irritation of the skin if applied prior to wetting the relevant areas. The rule is always read the manufacturer's recommendations.

Stage 3 – It is important that you always apply an appropriate cleansing agent to the areas for washing. The type of agent will be determined by the nature of the intended intervention:

- invasive/surgical
- antiseptic
- social.

It is not necessary to apply excessive amounts of the cleansing solution and the manufacturer's recommendations should always be followed.

Stage 4 – It is important that you wash all areas to be cleansed/decontaminated using an approved method and time period:

- social – minimum 15 seconds – hands and wrists;
- antiseptic – minimum 30 seconds – hands, wrists and up to mid forearm;
- invasive/surgical – minimum 2 minutes – hands, wrists and up to elbow.

Stage 5 – It is important that you rinse all areas washed until all trace of the cleansing agent has gone. Failure to do this may lead to skin irritation resulting from traces of the cleansing agent being left on your skin. In addition, where traces of the cleansing agent are left on the skin this may serve to facilitate bacterial re-colonisation.

Stage 6 – It is important to thoroughly dry all of the areas washed using:

- sterile hand towels for invasive/surgical interventions;
- sterile or disposable hand towels depending upon the nature of the intervention to be made;
- disposable hand towels or hot air blowers for social interventions.

The adoption of a biopsychosocial approach (*see* List 4.2) would serve to reduce the risks of such ethical and human rights breeches; for example, the concept of partnerships (Bleker 2000), where patients and clients are actively encouraged to become an integral part of their healthcare (*see* List 4.2, Points 3, 4, 7 and 8). When considered in the light of ever increasing rates of healthcare-acquired infections, such partnerships would seem to be particularly relevant from the perspective of self-preservation at the very least. Further, the adoption of a biopsychosocial approach would serve to facilitate enhanced self-awareness among health and social care professionals (*see* List 4.2, Points 1, 2, 4 and 6).

At this point go back and read through Tables 4.1 and 4.2. Then think about the differences that exist between biomedical and biopsychosocial approaches to standard precautions.

Once you've completed that, think about what aspects of your practice equate to a biopsychosocial approach and your adoption of standard precautions.

Take some time to reflect upon the chain of infection (*see* List 4.3). Do you feel it is consistent with a biomedical or biopsychosocial approach?

How valid and reliable do you feel the chain of infection is?

Because the current chain of infection (*see* List 4.3) is biomedical in its orientation and, in the absence of any empirical findings to substantiate it as a holistic and rigorous measure capable of contributing to long-term reductions in healthcare-acquired infections, it must be concluded that the chain of infection is neither valid nor reliable. Subsequently the chain of infection is of little practical value in making a useful contribution to reducing rates of both non-adherence to standard precautions and healthcare-acquired infections. At best such models are always tenuous in their ability to achieve what they purport to because they are developed by health and social care professionals who consistently demonstrate an amazing propensity for being susceptible to dissonance effects (*see* Explanation box 4.3), cognitively economic thinking (*see* Explanation box 4.1) and unrealistically optimistic beliefs (*see* Explanation box 4.2) in failing to recognise the necessity of adopting a biopsychosocial approach (*see* List 4.2).

How do you feel about the chain of infection?

What do you think could be done to develop the chain of infection to make it more reflective of a biopsychosocial approach?

How would making the chain of infection more biopsychosocial enhance its validity and reliability?

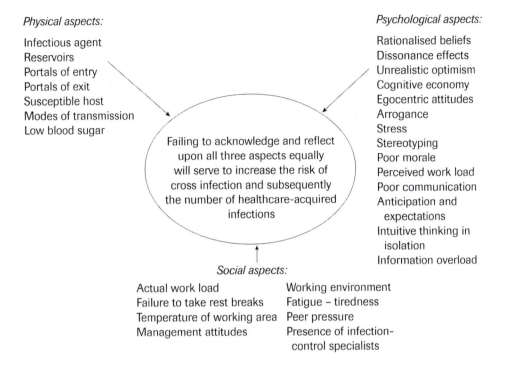

Physical aspects:

Infectious agent
Reservoirs
Portals of entry
Portals of exit
Susceptible host
Modes of transmission
Low blood sugar

Failing to acknowledge and reflect upon all three aspects equally will serve to increase the risk of cross infection and subsequently the number of healthcare-acquired infections

Psychological aspects:

Rationalised beliefs
Dissonance effects
Unrealistic optimism
Cognitive economy
Egocentric attitudes
Arrogance
Stress
Stereotyping
Poor morale
Perceived work load
Poor communication
Anticipation and
  expectations
Intuitive thinking in
  isolation
Information overload

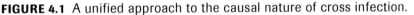

Social aspects:

Actual work load
Failure to take rest breaks
Temperature of working area
Management attitudes

Working environment
Fatigue – tiredness
Peer pressure
Presence of infection-
  control specialists

FIGURE 4.1 A unified approach to the causal nature of cross infection.

The chain of infection needs to be redefined to reflect a biopsychosocial approach. Although physical aspects do contribute, they are not the single cause of cross infection as the current chain of infection (*see* List 4.3) and biomedical approach (*see* List 4.1) would have us believe. Cross-infection rates will always be influenced by biopsychosocial (physical, psychological and social) factors (*see* List 4.2, Figure 4.1) and none can be held responsible in isolation for the transmission of infection.

Psychological factors that influence an individual's thinking will have a dominant influence over physical and social factors. For example, psychological factors such as cognitive dissonance (*see* Explanation box 4.3), cognitive economy (*see* Explanation box 4.1) and unrealistic optimism (*see* Explanation box 4.2) will determine the degree to which the individual adheres to standard precautions (Elliott 2003a). Therefore, the way an individual thinks about standard precautions will have dominance over physical factors (the availability of hand hygiene facilities) and social factors (the environment). The way an individual thinks about hand hygiene will be a combination of their attitudes towards the importance of undertaking such, and their beliefs about the consequences to themselves (not patients, clients or their colleagues) if they fail to adopt hand hygiene appropriately (*see* List 4.4). If an individual's attitude (way of thinking) causes them to ascribe hand hygiene as being of low importance and they hold a belief (accepted as truth) that there will be no consequences for failing to adopt appropriate hand hygiene, the combination of their attitude and belief will inevitably result in non-adherence – irrespective of what physical and social factors are present.

Inevitably, if adherence to standard precautions is to be improved on a consistent basis, a biopsychosocial approach must be adopted (*see* List 4.2, Table 4.2). Health and social care professionals and their employers must stop adopting a biomedical approach (*see* List 4.1, Table 4.1) and promoting the use of invalid and unreliable models (*see* List 4.3) if rising rates of healthcare-acquired infections are to be checked.

REFLECTION EXERCISE 4.6

What have you learnt about biomedical and biopsychosocial approaches in relation to infection control and the adoption of standard precautions?

In what ways will your infection control practice change having read this chapter?

CONCLUSION

This chapter has highlighted the importance of taking a biopsychosocial approach to the application of standard precautions and clearly shown that within infection control practice as a whole there will always be physical or physiological, psychological and social issues that must be acknowledged and dealt with in a unified way if infection control is to have maximum effect.

REFERENCES

Bleker O. Treat patients as you would like to be treated yourself. *BMJ*. 2000; **320**: 117.

Elliott P. Handwashing practice in nurse education. *Prof Nurse*. 1996; **11**(6): 359–60.

Elliott P. Recognising the psychosocial issues involved in hand hygiene. *J R Soc Promo Health*. 2003a; **123**(2): 88–94.

Elliott P. Failing to adopt a patient-centred approach: a multi-professional problem. *BMJ* (electronic responses); 2003b. Available at: www.bmj.com/cgi/eletters/326/7402/0#33297 (accessed 25 Nov 2008).

Elliott P, BVS Training. *Effective Hand Hygiene* (DVD/training pack). London: BVS Training; 2005. Available at: www.bvs.co.uk/index.asp (accessed 25 Nov 2008).

Festinger L. Cognitive dissonance. *Sci Am*. 1962; **207**: 93–102.

O'Dowd A. Nurses criticise poor hygiene practice among theatre staff. *Nurs Times.* 2006; **102**(16): 4.

Ogden J. *Health Psychology: a textbook.* 4th ed. Maidenhead: Open University Press/ McGraw-Hill Education; 2007.

Roper N, Logan W, Tierney A. *The Roper-Logan-Tierney Model of Nursing: based on activities of living.* London: Churchill Livingstone; 2000.

Roth I, Frisby J. *Perception and Representation: a cognitive approach.* Milton Keynes: Open University; 1992.

Sampson F. *Blackstone's Police Manual Volume 1: crime.* Oxford: Oxford University Press; 2006.

Seedhouse D. *Ethics: the heart of healthcare.* 2nd ed. Chichester: John Wiley and Sons; 1998.

Taylor A. Global governance, international health law and WHO: looking towards the future. *Bull World Health Organ.* 2002; **80**: 975–80.

Wilkinson R, Caulfield H. *The Human Rights Act: a practical guide for nurses.* Chichester: John Wiley; 2001.

CHAPTER 5

Psychosocial theories and approaches in perspective

This chapter will individually present a number of psychosocial theories and approaches (*see* Figure 5.1). The aim in presenting them this way is to facilitate understanding. However, the information in Figure 5.1 should be seen as offering examples rather than being mutually exclusive. As with previous

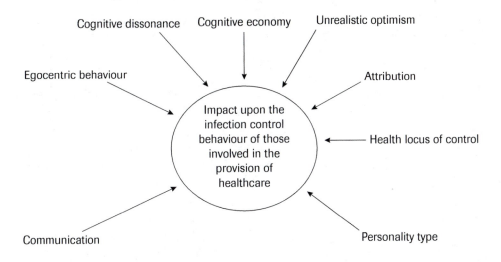

NB: The information identified above should not be seen as being mutually exclusive but rather as offering examples.

FIGURE 5.1 Psychosocial theories and related approaches influencing infection control behaviour.

chapters, the discussion will be interspaced with a series of reflection exercises aimed at further enhancing your understanding.

COGNITIVE DISSONANCE

Cognitive dissonance (*see* Explanation box 5.1) proposes that at a cognitive level, individuals will strive to make two or more things consistent that would not normally be so (Morrison and Bennett 2006).

EXPLANATION BOX 5.1 COGNITIVE DISSONANCE (FESTINGER 1962)

The concept of cognitive dissonance was originally identified by Festinger (1962), where he proposed that, at a psychological level, the individual will strive to make consistent two or more things that would not naturally be so. In simple terms, dissonance effects are when an individual generates excuses to justify their previous behaviour or behaviour they wish or intend to carry out. Hand hygiene is a good example, where the individual understands its importance in reducing cross infection, yet fails to adequately follow the hand hygiene process. Thus the individual experiences conflict between knowing what they should do and what they actually do or want to do.

Such conflict would be manifest as stress in the individual and in an attempt to reduce such stress the individual will generate an excuse or reason for failing to follow the hand hygiene process. Such an excuse may be blamed on time, work load or an irrational belief that meeting other's needs must take priority.

This means that when an individual is confronted with a situation where they know what they should do, but this is in opposition with what they want to do or have done, the individual will experience psychological conflict. Such conflict would be manifested in their behaviour in a variety of ways; for example, as stress, agitation, irritability, mood swings, arrogance, egocentrism or a combination of all these.

REFLECTION EXERCISE 5.1

Within your own practice, can you think of any situations where you knew what you should do but what you actually did was in opposition?

Take some time to think about how that situation made you feel. You may also want to think about what effects your behaviour had upon others. An example might be that after using the bathroom you simply rinsed your hands under running water as opposed to knowing full well that you should have adopted hand hygiene (*see* List 5.1).

LIST 5.1 HAND HYGIENE PROCESS (ELLIOTT 2003)

Stage 1 – It is vital that you recognise the need to undertake hand hygiene. This is probably the most important stage within the process because if you fail to recognise situations where you need to adopt formal hand hygiene as opposed to using cleansing gels, then the remainder of the process will at worst not occur and at best occur intermittently. Either way the risk of cross infection will be increased.

Stage 2 – It is important that you thoroughly wet all areas to be washed with running water. Failure do this may lead to you experiencing skin problems because some cleansing agents can cause irritation of the skin if applied prior to wetting the relevant areas. The rule is always read the manufacturer's recommendations.

Stage 3 – It is important that you always apply an appropriate cleansing agent to the areas for washing. The type of agent will be determined by the nature of the intended intervention:
- invasive/surgical
- antiseptic
- social.

It is not necessary to apply excessive amounts of the cleansing solution and the manufacturer's recommendations should always be followed.

Stage 4 – It is important that you wash, using running water, the areas to be cleansed/decontaminated using an approved method and time period:
- social – minimum 15 seconds – hands and wrists;
- antiseptic – minimum 30 seconds – hands, wrists and up to mid forearm;
- invasive/surgical – minimum 2 minutes – hands, wrists and up to elbow.

Stage 5 – It is important that you rinse all areas washed until all trace of the cleansing agent has gone. Failure to do this may lead to skin irritation resulting from traces of the cleansing agent being left on your skin. In addition, where traces of the cleansing agent are left on the skin this may serve to facilitate bacterial re-colonisation.

Stage 6 – It is important to thoroughly dry all of the areas washed using:

- sterile hand towels for invasive/surgical interventions;
- sterile or disposable hand towels depending upon the nature of the intervention to be made;
- disposable hand towels or hot air blowers for social interventions.

It is important that you were absolutely honest when undertaking Reflection exercise 5.1. Within healthcare, the cutting of corners where infection control is concerned occurs on a regular basis, so if you feel you may not have been as honest as you should have been, you may want to repeat the exercise. The cutting of corners to make our lives easier is a trade off where we generate excuses to justify our actions. However, these excuses are dissonance-based (*see* Explanation box 5.1) and will result in dangerous practice. Below are three examples of dissonance effects applied to practice:

Example 1: A nurse or midwife understands the importance of changing gloves yet fails to do so and attempts to justify their behaviour through such excuses as 'I haven't got time to change my gloves between each individual I make contact with. I am much too busy trying to complete all the tasks allocated to me! Anyway, they aren't dirty; look – there is nothing on them.'

Example 2: In the case of a psychologist or social worker who fails to adopt hand hygiene, they may generate the excuse 'There's no need for me to worry about washing my hands as I do not make physical contact with my clients.' Yet the ability of an individual to cross infect is not restricted to direct physical contact with others.

Example 3: A medical practitioner is meticulous about their hand hygiene in preparing to undertake an invasive procedure within an operating department setting, but then fails to adopt the same meticulous approach when examining a postoperative wound in a ward setting. In such a case, when challenged about this they may generate the excuse that 'As the patient's wound has healed there is little risk of cross infection.' Whether or not a wound has healed the risk of cross infection will not be negated.

These examples illustrate one of Festinger's (1962) original points: that for the most part individuals are not rational, rather they rationalise. Clearly the rationalisations outlined above do not constitute rational thinking. In fact, where safe practice is concerned, they are completely irrational.

COGNITIVE ECONOMY

Cognitive economy (*see* Explanation box 5.2) is a process where individuals attempt to gain maximum output for minimum cognitive effort.

EXPLANATION BOX 5.2 COGNITIVE ECONOMY
(ROTH AND FRISBY 1992)

Cognitive economy is where an individual has become context-specific or tunnel-visioned in their perception of what is occurring around them and will fail to take into account the wider implications of their behaviour. For example, instead of being patient-centred, the individual will become task-orientated towards achieving a set of goals that will meet their own needs at the expense of everything else and the needs of others.

Example: In the case of standard precautions, the individual will be context-specific towards achieving their allocated work load and as a result of this may:
- fail to change their gloves between interventions;
- fail to undertake or to fully follow the hand hygiene process;
- fail to ensure that they have removed all the equipment they used following completion of a procedure.

As Reason (1998 p. 44) points out, 'humans, if given the choice, would prefer to act as context-specific pattern recognisers rather that attempting to calculate or optimize.' In other words, individuals prefer to be tunnel-visioned and task-orientated as opposed to considering the wider context and being person-centred. Why? Because the former requires less cognitive effort. Subsequently, the individual will focus upon a set of goals that are important to them, but may not be consistent with the needs of patients or clients, which is detrimental to safe practice and will be more in tune with a biomedical approach (*see* List 5.2). Below are two examples of a cognitively economic perspective (*see* Explanation box 5.2):

Example 1: Where an individual believes that meeting a patient or client's physical needs in isolation will be sufficient to promote health and wellbeing. Such a belief is cognitively economic because they fail to recognise that psychological and social needs also affect an individual's health and wellbeing.

Example 2: Where health and social care professionals use the term 'hand washing' as opposed to 'hand hygiene'. Using the term 'hand washing' will lead to a focus on the washing aspects of the hand hygiene process in isolation (*see* List 5.1), thus significantly increasing the potential for other aspects of the process to be neglected or completely ignored.

LIST 5.2 RELATING THE BIOMEDICAL MODEL TO INFECTION CONTROL

This model (Elliott and BVS Training 2005) assumes that:

1 The concepts of health and illness are seen to exist separately.
   Infection control example: Healthcare-acquired infection and the interventions made by health and social care professionals are seen as existing in isolation; they are not perceived as impacting upon each other.

2 Disease or infection is external to the body and is not the result of an individual's behaviour.
   Infection control example: The behaviour of health and social care professionals has no impact upon the risk of cross infection.

3 Individuals should have no control over or involvement with what happens to them regarding their health and wellbeing.
   Infection control example: Patients and clients have no right to question or challenge health and social care professionals even though the patient or client may have contracted a healthcare-acquired infection through the health and social care professional's negligence as a result of their poor and inadequate adoption of standard precautions.

4 Individuals have no responsibility to ensure the maintenance of their own or others' health and wellbeing.
   Infection control example: Despite failing to adopt standard precautions, health and social care professionals are not responsible for the consequences of such a failure.

5 Although it is acknowledged they exist, the mind and body are perceived as being separate with neither having consequences for the other.
   Infection control example: A health and social care professional who is experiencing stress will demonstrate a greater propensity towards becoming cognitively economic (*see* Explanation box 5.2) and unrealistically optimistic (*see* Explanation box 5.3) in their perception of the importance of standard precautions. Despite this, there will be no impact upon their behaviour; therefore, a failure to carry out standard precautions according to a biomedical perspective is not a consequence of the way a health or social care professional thinks but simply a physical action.

6 Psychosocial factors have no part to play and healthcare intervention should centre around the physical aspects in isolation.
   Infection control example: Healthcare-acquired infection has nothing to do with how health and social care professionals think or the social context within which they are practising. Cross infection is simply a consequence of the physical factors, such as the cleanliness of equipment, the environment or staff uniforms/work clothing.

7 Health and social care professionals are knowledgeable experts who always know best.
   Infection control example: Attitudes such as 'I am safe', 'I am competent', 'I know what I am doing' or 'I am an expert' are all indicative of dissonance-based thinking (*see* Explanation box 5.1) and a cognitively economic perspective (*see* Explanation box 5.2) towards their ability to carry out consistent safe infection control practice. However, terms such as 'safe', 'competent' and 'expert' are all spurious in nature and are reflective of an egocentric and conceited self-perception, which serves to precipitate unsafe infection-control behaviour.

8 Patients and clients cease to have their own identity. Rather they become stereotyped or labelled by health and social care professionals.
   Infection control example: Patients and clients who contract a healthcare-acquired infection may be seen as the health problem they present within isolation, as opposed to a person in their own right. For example, an individual with MRSA loses the right to be seen as a person, and becomes an entity. This entity principle has particular relevance when a patient or client having contracted a healthcare-acquired infection is placed in a side room, becomes perceived as dirty and are then forgotten – out of sight and out of mind!

9 It is acceptable to ridicule a patient or client when they fail to conform to the assumptions, expectations or requirements of health and social care professionals.
   Infection control example: Patients and clients who experience a healthcare-acquired infection become stigmatised by health and social care professionals who may originally have been responsible for them contracting an infection in the first place. As a result of such they are perceived as failing to conform with the expectations of those health and social care professionals.

NB: The above should not be seen as being mutually exclusive, but rather as providing a perspective.

Try to think of examples where you may have been cognitively economic with regard to your infection control practice. When reflecting upon this, you may find it helpful to think of cognitive economy as cutting corners to achieve what you want.

Where have you cut corners regarding your adoption of standard precautions?

In what ways do you think this placed you and others at risk of cross infection?

UNREALISTIC OPTIMISM

Unrealistic optimism (*see* Explanation box 5.3) is a process where individuals behave in ways that put themselves and others at risk.

EXPLANATION BOX 5.3 UNREALISTIC OPTIMISM (OGDEN 2007)

Unrealistic optimism is where a health or social care professional becomes unrealistically optimistic regarding risky situations they place themselves and others in as a result of behaviour that constitutes unsafe infection control practice in the form of failing to undertake standard precautions or through failing to follow the hand hygiene process.

Unrealistic optimism can be facilitated through lack of personal experience. For example, a health or social care professional who has no prior experience of a patient's or client's health being directly influenced by their failure to adopt appropriate standard precautions will likely believe two things (Elliott 2003):

1 There is no risk, or the risk of cross infecting others is so insignificant that it simply does not matter.

2 Even if there is a risk it will not happen to them. That is, even if the individual involved in healthcare does cross infect others they will rationalise that is was not their fault (*see* Explanation box 5.1) or they will not be found out and held responsible and therefore, who cares?

Unrealistic optimism has close links with cognitive dissonance (*see* Explanation box 5.1) because they are both ways in which an individual can justify their unsafe behaviour. The difference is that with cognitive dissonance the individual generates irrational excuses, whereas with unrealistic optimism the individual has a distorted belief of the risks involved in carrying out certain types of behaviour. Below are two examples of distorted beliefs as a result of unrealistic optimism:

Example 1: The 'It will not happen to me' syndrome (Elliott 2003) where the individual believes that undertaking a given behaviour will not produce negative consequences for them. In the case of hand hygiene, such a distorted belief may centre around an understanding that the need to dry the hands thoroughly is not as important as undertaking the washing component of the hand hygiene process (*see* List 5.1).

Example 2: Individuals who have no personal experience of standard precautions being applied or the consequences of failing to apply them will be highly susceptible to unrealistic optimism. Such individuals may be administrators, psychologists, social workers, senior management and educationalists. These individuals may be unrealistically optimistic regarding the risks associated with non-adherence to standard precautions because they hold dissonance-based beliefs about their susceptibility to cross infection. For example:

➤ the senior manager or administrator who believes that because they do not go near areas where there are patients with infections they are not at risk and as such do not need to adopt appropriate standard precautions;

➤ the psychologist or social worker who believes that only patients in hospital catch harmful infections and as such do not need to adopt appropriate standard precautions such as hand hygiene when clients visit them;

➤ educationalists who believe that because they do not work in areas where infected patients or clients are present they will not be at risk of catching anything and as such do not need to adopt appropriate standard precautions.

REFLECTION EXERCISE 5.3

Identify situations where you have been unrealistically optimistic regarding the risk you have placed yourself or others at in relation to your adoption of standard precautions.

HEALTH LOCUS OF CONTROL

EXPLANATION BOX 5.4 HEALTH LOCUS OF CONTROL (ADAMS
AND BROMLEY 1998; WALLSTON AND WALLSTON 1982)

Locus of control consists of two dimensions:

1 Internal: This is the partnership between the patient or client and the healthcare worker, whether it be professional, administrative, managerial or ancillary. Such partnerships reflect the provision of information, non-judgemental attitudes and the right to ask questions without fear of ridicule and retribution. Such an approach is reflective of a biopsychosocial perspective (*see* List 5.3).
   Example: With regard to standard precautions, patients and clients have the right to have their questions answered in order for them to make informed choices as to whether they wish to comply with the advice given by healthcare workers.
2 External: This is where the patient or client is expected to be unquestioning, compliant and submissive to the demands of healthcare workers. Such an approach is reflective of a biomedical perspective (*see* List 5.2).
   Example: With regard to standard precautions, patients and clients are denied the opportunity to ensure that these are appropriately applied within the context of their healthcare experience.

Internal locus of control is where an individual believes they have the power to influence outcomes. Such an approach is consistent with a biopsychosocial and person-centred approaches where a partnership exists between the patient or client and healthcare workers, whether they are professional, managerial, administrative or ancillary.

Example: With regard to infection control, patients and clients should feel able to challenge professionals about using standard precautions with the expectation that their challenge will be received in a professional manner in accordance with Article 10 of the Human Rights Act (1998), the right 'to hold opinions and receive and impart information' (Wilkinson and Caulfield 2001 p. 36) and that an appropriate response will be given.

LIST 5.3 RELATING THE BIOPSYCHOSOCIAL
MODEL TO INFECTION CONTROL

This model (Elliott and BVS Training 2005) assumes that:

1   The concepts of health and illness are perceived as coexisting on a
    continuum.
    Infection control example: Contracting a healthcare-acquired infection will
    impact upon different individuals' life spans and ability to carry out their
    activities of daily living (Roper, Logan and Tierney 2000) in fundamentally
    different ways.

2   Infection can be internal or external to the body and may be the result of an
    individual's health behaviour.
    Infection control example: An internal cause of infection may be the result
    of a patient or client's behaviour. An external cause of infection may be the
    result of the behaviour of health and social care professionals – both of
    which may lead to the contracting of a healthcare-acquired infection.

3   Patients and clients should be offered the opportunity to be actively involved
    in the decision-making process with regard to their health and wellbeing.
    Infection control example: Patients and clients should be actively encouraged
    to challenge and question the judgements and decisions of health and social
    care professionals regarding the degree to which they apply the principles
    of safe infection control practice. If a health and social care professional fails
    to facilitate such, they may well find themselves in contravention of a patient
    or client's human rights.

4   Individuals should accept responsibility for their own health behaviour.
    Infection control example: Health and social care professionals must accept
    responsibility for their health behaviour from two standpoints:
    ● accepting responsibility for the quality and standard of their infection
      control practice;
    ● accepting responsibility for their own health and wellbeing. For
      example, if they are unwell and aware that they may be potentially
      infectious then they should act in an appropriate professional manner.

5   The physical, psychological and social aspects that make up an individual
    coexist, with each having the potential to impact upon the other.
    Infection control example: Failing to adopt standard precautions will have
    physical, psychological and social consequences for health and social care
    professionals, patients and clients and for society as a whole.

6   Psychosocial factors carry equal importance to physical factors with regard
    to healthcare intervention.
    Infection control example: Where the adoption of standard precautions are

concerned, health and social care professionals must recognise that they will have physical, psychological and social implications for patients and clients.

7   Patients and clients may have a greater knowledge of their health problem than the health and social care professionals.
    Infection control example: Health and social care professionals should work in partnership with patients and clients with the aim of ensuring that standard precautions occur on a consistent basis.

8   Patients and clients should be empowered towards retaining their own identity whilst receiving healthcare intervention.
    Infection control example: Facilitating an individual towards retaining their own identity as opposed to conditioning/categorising them into the patient role will empower them towards questioning and challenging poor infection-control practice when it occurs.

9   If health and social care professionals fail to recognise the necessity of a biopsychosocial approach, this can cause life-span consequences for patients and clients.
    Infection control example: The appropriate adoption of standard precautions by health and social care professionals has important implications regarding the future physical, psychological and social aspects of an individual's life span.

External locus of control is where an individual believes they have little power to influence what will happen to them. Such an approach is consistent with biomedical and task-orientated approaches (*see* List 5.2) where the patient or client is at the mercy of health and social care professionals. For example, with regard to the potential for contracting MRSA, a person admitted to a healthcare establishment would be powerless to control the degree of risk they would be exposed to from health and social care professionals' failure to adopt standard precautions.

REFLECTION EXERCISE 5.4

In considering the above, have you ever been challenged about your infection-control practice?

If you have, how did you feel about being challenged and how did you react to the person challenging you?

If you have never been challenged about your infection-control practice, please think about why that was. In reflecting upon this, you might like to consider if it was because the patient or client was frightened to challenge you in case the subsequent quality of care you gave them declined and they feared you might cause them harm (Salmon 2000).

ATTRIBUTION

Attribution (Adams and Bromley 1998; Huffman, Vernoy and Vernoy 2000) is related to how individuals make judgements of others' behaviour based upon minimal and very dubious evidence. Yet this is something that health and social care professionals are extremely good at and do so without any consideration of the consequences of their judgements. For example, medical practitioners have suffered much ridicule regarding their being causal agents for cross infection by the media and other health and social care professionals (Howlett 2005; Lister 2004; Miller *et al.* 2003; Stuttaford 2004). However, in making such judgements, which may be subject to discrimination resulting from dissonance effects (Explanation box 5.1), cognitive economy (Explanation box 5.2) and unrealistic optimism (Explanation box 5.3), individuals fail to recognise that they may be just as guilty of being causal agents of cross infection.

Much has and continues to be made about the importance of adopting appropriate hand hygiene within all areas of society and there are many who readily make judgements about the quality of others' hand hygiene behaviour. Yet how many of those who are only too ready to criticise and attribute cause of cross infection to others could honestly state that they themselves have always adopted appropriate hand hygiene when they should have? Interestingly, some years back I was privileged to be asked to speak at two major international infection control conferences. On both occasions, before I began my presentation, I asked all those present to raise their hands up if they had always washed their hands when they knew they should have. Within one group of delegates not one individual raised their hand, and in the other group the number was minimal. In addition, whilst at these conferences and with the consent of the conference organisers, I carried out a survey using a five-point Likert Scale (*see* List 5.4).

LIST 5.4 PARTICIPANT QUESTIONNAIRE

Code Number   Age: Gender: Male/Female

Occupation: Microbiologist/Infection Control Nurse/Other ....

PLEASE DO NOT IDENTIFY YOURSELF IN ANY OTHER WAY THAN THAT REQUESTED ABOVE

Statements	Strongly Agree	Agree	Undecided	Disagree	Strongly Disagree
1 Microbiologists are essential to the infection control team					
2 The infection control team is multi-professional enough					
3 Psychologists would be a useful edition to the team					
4 Nurses are important members of the infection control team					
5 Doctors are less important to the team than nurses					
6 Educationalists would make a useful contribution to the infection-control team					
7 Expanding the multi-professional membership of the team would be a bad thing					
8 Infection-control nurses and microbiologists need the help of other professional disciplines in reducing cross infection					
9 Education is the best method of changing people's infection-control behaviour					
10 Health psychologists could contribute to reducing cross-infection rates					
11 Infection-control nurses and microbiologists understand the psychosocial issues involved in poor infection-control practice					

Statements	Strongly Agree	Agree	Undecided	Disagree	Strongly Disagree
12 Psychosocial issues in infection control; what a load of rubbish!					
13 Infection control should be left to infection-control nurses who know what they are doing					
14 Who needs infection-control nurses? Microbiologists can do the job just as well.					
15 The infection-control team would benefit from having a more multi-professional membership					
16 Healthcare educators spend too little time in the clinical setting to be worthy of a place on the infection-control team					
17 Potential and actual recipients of healthcare would be a welcome addition as members of the infection-control team					
18 Infection-control nurses and microbiologists are losing the fight against reducing cross infection					
19 I always adhere to standard precautions					
20 Multi-professional approaches towards reducing cross-infection rates are a waste of time					
21 Health and occupational psychologists understand the dangers of cross infection					
22 Compliance with safe infection-control practice is best achieved through the use of policies and procedures					

(*continued*)

Statements	Strongly Agree	Agree	Undecided	Disagree	Strongly Disagree
23 I feel the underlying cause of non-adherence to infection-control practice is psychosocial					
24 Poor infection-control practice is about the way people think and not what they do					
25 Psychologists deal with the way people think, which has nothing to do with reducing cross infection					
26 Infection-control specialists have a greater understanding of the issues involved in preventing cross infection than others involved in the provision of healthcare					
27 Reducing cross-infection rates is about changing people's attitudes					
28 The infection-control team needs to expand its membership if it is ever to deal with the true nature of poor infection-control practice					
29 Health and occupational psychologists have a better understanding of work-related behaviour change. They would therefore make a valuable contribution to the infection-control team					
30 Enforced prescriptive rules ensure compliance; multi-disciplinary working does not					
31 No one else understands infection control better than infection-control specialists					
32 The underlying nature of non-adherence to infection-control practice is psychosocial					

Statements	Strongly Agree	Agree	Undecided	Disagree	Strongly Disagree
33 A less multi-disciplinary approach to infection control would help to reduce the risk of cross infection					
34 Multi-professional approaches to controlling the spread of infection are a waste of time					
35 Doctors are the principal cause of cross infection					
36 Nurses are the principal cause of cross infection					
37 Professions allied to medicine are the principal cause of cross infection					
38 Making the infection-control team more multi-disciplinary is essential in reducing cross infection in the future					
39 Psychologists should become full-time members of the infection-control team					
40 Healthcare educators should become full-time members of the infection-control team					
41 Porters, cleaners and other ancillary staff are the principal cause of cross infection					
42 Recipients of healthcare intervention are the principal cause of cross infection					
43 As a practitioner/expert in my field I always know what is right where infection control is concerned					
44 Infection control is everyone's responsibility and not just that of the infection-control specialists					

(*continued*)

Statements	Strongly Agree	Agree	Undecided	Disagree	Strongly Disagree
45 It would be an impossible task to increase the multi-disciplinary membership of the infection control team					
46 Reducing hospital-acquired infection does not require the input of health educators and psychologists despite the psychosocial nature of the problem					
47 The input of psychologists and educators within the community is not necessary because the prevalence of cross infection is less than in the acute setting					

48 In the space below, please comment on how you feel about involving health/occupational psychologists and healthcare educators as members of the infection-control team:

I have not provided a quantitative analysis for this survey, but below are some qualitative findings:

Some statements and specific narrative responses

Statement 21: Health and occupational psychologists understand the dangers of cross infection.

Response: Women are much better at infection control than men.

Statement 24: Poor infection-control practice is about the way people think and not what they do.

Response: No! They are too busy and we also don't have enough wash basins.

Statement 27: Reducing cross infection is about changing people's attitudes.

Response: Disagree. It's about recruiting more nurses.

Statement 31: No one else understands infection control better than infection-control specialists.

Response: Women particularly have a 'nose' for hygiene.

Some other narrative comments:

➤ Microbiology is the basis of all infection;

➤ A psychologist is of no use in an infection-control team;

➤ In my experience, educators know very little about infection control.

The above responses clearly attribute dissonance-based and cognitively economic perspectives towards infection control.

Attributing cause is a form of defence mechanism where individuals attempt to divert blame away from themselves. Further, it is based upon an egocentric and dissonance-based belief that their judgements of others are correct.

REFLECTION EXERCISE 5.5

Try and think of any situations where you or those around you may have attempted to attribute cause with regard to cross infection.

In reflecting upon this, consider how ethical attributing the cause of cross infection is when the person doing the attributing may be just as guilty.

EGOCENTRIC BEHAVIOUR

Egocentric behaviour (Atkinson *et al.* 2000; Ogden 2007) may be described as self-centred and self-orientated behaviour without consideration of others and generally tends to be ascribed to the kinds of behaviour that might be observed in young children. However, such egocentric behaviour is not confined to children, but also can be observed in the behaviour of adults.

Example: Where a health or social care professional believes that others should clear up after them because they think their appointment or role excuses them from having to do so themselves.

COMMUNICATION

Communication (Potter and Perry 2001), where adherence to standard precautions is concerned, is a fundamental aspect of ensuring that safe practice is undertaken. Individuals who always believe what their peers tell them as being correct or that observation of others is a sound method of judging behaviour are running the risk of practising in an unsafe manner. In reality, the drawing of intuitive or peer-based inferences (Elliott 2003) from observing another's behaviour can lead to problems of interpretation. The dangers of believing that practice based upon accepting absolutely what our peers tell us or intuitively interpreting what we observe in others as correct are highlighted within the two explanations below:

Danger 1: Where information is being passed from one individual to another it is generally assumed that the information being given is accurate. However, to make such an assumption is unrealistically optimistic (*see* Explanation box 5.3) because when we communicate with each other we only impart information that we believe is relevant and important for others to know. Unfortunately, there can be a significant difference between what we believe others should know and what they actually need to know. Such a disparity can lead to unsafe practice.

Danger 2: When we witness an event there is always the potential for misinterpretation because what we interpret from our observation of a given event may not be a true reflection of what has actually happened. Where observation is concerned we will always interpret what we see and hear according to our own past experience, expectations and pre-conceived ideas. Thus interpretation through observation of what our peers do is highly suspect and should always be questioned.

REFLECTION EXERCISE 5.6

Think about what your colleagues have said to you about standard precautions in the past or your observation of their undertaking standard precautions.
In reflecting upon the above:
1 Did what your colleagues say to you about standard precautions differ from their adoption of them?
2 If there was a contradiction between what your colleagues said and did regarding standard precautions, how did that make you feel?
3 Does listening to what colleagues tell you and observing what they do always reflect safe practice?
4 Where listening to others and observing their practice is concerned, what will you do in future?

PERSONALITY

Personality (Atkinson *et al.* 2000) can offer a causal reason for the reasons health and social care professionals fail to adopt standard precautions. Such a premise can be approached from three perspectives: personality type, personality factors and structure of personality.

Personality type

The personality type approach is where we can draw a distinction between types A and B personalities (*see* List 5.5) with the former being less likely to adhere to standard precautions than the latter.

LIST 5.5 TYPE A AND TYPE B PERSONALITY CHARACTERISTICS

Type A	Type B
Exacting in their expectations of others	More reflective
Controlling and hates losing	Creative
Fastidious	Imaginative
Precise in how something should be undertaken	Greater degree of patience
A need to prevail	More able to relax
Achieve more in less time	Able to pace themselves more easily
Task-orientated	Less ambitious
Propensity towards unprovoked anger, hostility and unpredictable aggression	Less irritable
Competitive and impatient	Greater awareness of their limitations
Always rushing and ambitious	Socially more adept
Having a desire for recognition	Rarely irritated by events or situations
Constantly feeling a need to achieve	More effective critical thinkers
Cynical and critical of others	Methodical
Ruthless in how their goals are achieved	Less time-orientated
Rapid speech	More effective communicators
There is never enough time	Greater acceptance of others
Irritable, restless and hates having their time wasted.	More of a team player
Tendency to underestimate	
Likes to dominate and interrupt	

In considering this further, an individual whose behaviour reflects Type A characteristics (*see* List 5.5) will have a greater propensity towards adopting a biomedical approach (*see* List 5.2), as they are likely to be task-orientated and less likely to adhere to standard precautions. In contrast, an individual's behaviour which reflects Type B characteristics (*see* List 5.5) will have a greater propensity towards adopting a biopsychosocial approach (*see* List 5.3), as they are person-centred and will be more likely to adhere to standard precautions. This is because Type A personalities will be more susceptible to the effects of cognitive dissonance (*see* Explanation box 5.1), cognitive economy (*see* Explanation box 5.2) and unrealistic optimism (*see* Explanation box 5.3). Furthermore, Type A personalities will be more orientated towards adopting an external locus of control (*see* Explanation box 5.4). However, Type B personalities are likely to have a broader perspective. For example, within the context of the thinking/practice continuum (*see* Table 5.1) Type A personalities' thinking will be predisposed to occur at Levels 4, 5 or 6; whereas Type B personalities' thinking will be predisposed to utilising all levels of the continuum or those levels that are most appropriate at any given moment.

TABLE 5.1 Thinking/practice continuum

Levels	Definition
Level 1: Research-based thinking	Individual validates their practice through published research
Level 2: Evidence-based thinking	Individual validates their practice through clinical evidence
Level 3: Reflective thinking	Individual validates their practice through reflecting on their and others' actions
Level 4: System-supported thinking	Individual validates their practice through information provided by machinery/diagnostic aids
Level 5: Peer-generated thinking	Individual validates their practice based upon what their peers/colleagues tell them
Level 6: Intuitive thinking	Individual validates their practice according to their own subjective attitudes and beliefs

(Adapted from Hamm cited in Dowie and Elstein 1996)

Safe practice will be facilitated if an individual's thinking reflects a flow between all levels of the above continuum.

Example 1: An individual whose thinking occurs at one level in isolation within the continuum and presents as a Type A personality (*see* List 5.5) will be unsafe in their adoption of standard precautions and particularly so when thinking occurs at levels 4, 5 or 6.

Example 2: An individual whose thinking encompasses all levels of the continuum and presents as a Type B personality (*see* List 5.5) will be more likely to adopt standard precautions in an appropriate way.

Personality factors (Eysenck in Blinkhorn 1981)

The personality factors approach presents a distinction between the stable and unstable dimensions of Eysenck's Personality Factors Model (*see* Figure 5.2). Within the context of this model, when the behaviour of a health and social care professional is reflective of those factors set out within the unstable dimension (*see* Figure 5.2) they will have a greater propensity towards adopting a biomedical approach (List 5.2), be task-orientated and be less likely to adopt standard precautions. However, when a health and social care professional's behaviour is reflective of those factors set out within the stable dimension (*see* Figure 5.2) they will have a greater propensity towards adopting a biopsychosocial approach (List 5.3), be person-centred and be more likely to adopt standard precautions in an appropriate way. This is because those factors identified within the unstable dimension are consistent

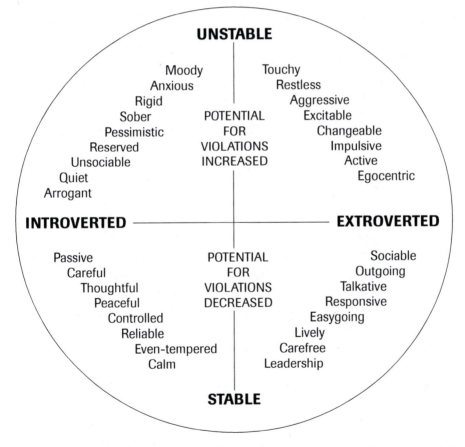

FIGURE 5.2 Linking Eysenck's personality factors model to the potential for infection control violations. Adapted from Atkinson RL *et al. Hilgard's Introduction to Psychology.* 13th ed. London: International Thomson Publishing; 2000.

with Type A characteristics (*see* List 5.5) and will be more susceptible to the effects of cognitive dissonance, cognitive economy, unrealistic optimism and function within the confines of an external locus of control. Therefore Type A characteristics (*see* List 5.5) and unstable personality factors (*see* Figure 5.2) will both enhance the risk of an individual becoming unsafe in practice. In contrast, Type B characteristics (*see* List 5.5) and stable personality factors (*see* Figure 5.2) will both enhance an individual's potential for safe practice.

However, it must not be assumed that personality types, characteristics or factors are absolutes; i.e. that an individual is either a Type A or Type B (*see* List 5.5), or exhibiting stable/unstable or introvert/extrovert personality characteristics (*see* Figure 5.2). To make such an assumption would be highly questionable. In reality, all are dynamic processes where individuals move between Type A or Type B, between stable/unstable or between introvert/extrovert characteristics. This is dependent upon a variety of reasons, which may include physical, psychological and social influences:

Physical	Psychological	Social
The environment	An individual's mood	Peer group
Time of day/night	Degree of stress experienced	Peer approval
Work load	Attitudes and beliefs	Quality of communication
Level of fatigue	Degree of safety and security felt	Quality of relationships

The above should not be seen as being mutually exclusive but as offering examples.

Structure of personality

The structure of personality is where a distinction between the id, the ego and the superego exists (*see* Figure 5.3). Within the context of this model, the health or social care professional who is task-orientated, unrealistically optimistic and cognitively economic will have the propensity to function primarily at the id level (*see* Figure 5.3). As such they will be egocentric in their singular orientation towards meeting their own needs as opposed to meeting the needs of patients or clients. For example, the health or social care professional who fails to recognise the wider consequences of not adhering to standard precautions because they are pleasure seeking (within the context of gaining satisfaction from completing their work load) even though this may be at the expense of protecting the patient or client from cross infection. Functioning at the id level will lead to the stereotyping of individuals according to the health problem; for example, identifying the patient by their condition, not their name: 'the appendix in bed 4' or 'the leg ulcer at number 29'. What I find interesting about

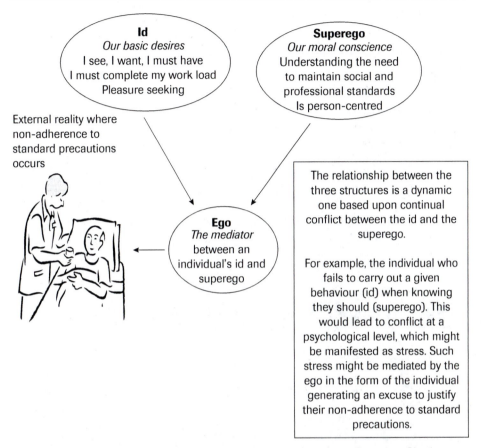

FIGURE 5.3 The structure of personality: id, ego, superego (Freud in Slack 1981).

such designations is that I have never seen an appendix in a bed! I have seen a person with or without an appendix in a bed but never just an appendix! In reality such designations are neither professional, ethical or appropriate. In contrast, the health or social care professional who recognises the need for a person-centred approach and understands the concept of continuing care and that patients and clients have biopsychosocial needs (Ogden 2007), will have the propensity to function at the superego level (*see* Figure 5.3).

There are two points which need to be made in consideration of the id and superego. Firstly, the processes of cognitive dissonance (*see* Explanation box 5.1), cognitive economy (*see* Explanation box 5.2) and unrealistic optimism (*see* Explanation box 5.3) will all enhance the potential for an individual to function at the id level. This is because all three processes are consistent with id level functioning in allowing an individual to justify the meeting of their own needs. Secondly, it is believed that the ego is responsible for mediating between the id and the superego. For example, 'I must complete my work load through task orientation and as such I may have to abandon undertaking standard precautions.' This is an id perspective. Alternatively, consider 'Although I need to complete my work load I must do this through being person-centred and the adoption of standard precautions as a means of protecting the patient from harm.' This is a superego perspective. If the health and social care professional were to recognise the id and superego perspectives, it would lead to psychological conflict, which might well be manifested as the feeling of stress. In order to resolve this stress, the health or social care professional's ego would have to mediate between the two perspectives. In order to allow mediation to occur and their stress to be resolved, the individual would generate dissonance-based excuses, which would then allow them to adopt and justify – without further conflict – either an id- or superego-based behaviour.

REFLECTION EXERCISE 5.7

1 With regards to the id and superego perspectives above, which should you choose?
2 In reflecting upon your own adoption of standard precautions, which perspective have you sometimes actually chosen?

In thinking about the two points above, it is important that you are honest with yourself. What you may find is that you have provided yourself with an example of where you knew that what you should do differed with what you actually did. You might then want to ask yourself the question 'How safe is my infection-control practice?'

CONCLUSION

I hope that you now have a better understanding of how psychosocial theories and approaches can influence everyday infection-control practice. In undertaking the reflection exercises I hope you have increased your understanding of how your own infection-control practice may have been affected by those theories and approaches.

REFERENCES

Adams B, Bromley B. *Psychology for Healthcare: key terms and concepts.* Macmillan: Basingstoke; 1998.

Atkinson RL, Atkinson RC, Smith E, *et al. Hilgard's Introduction to Psychology.* 13th ed. Harcourt College: London; 2000.

Elliott P. Recognising the psychosocial issues involved in hand hygiene. *J R Soc Promo Health.* 2003; **123**(2): 88–94.

Elliott P, BVS Training. *Effective Hand Hygiene* (DVD/training pack). London: BVS Training; 2005. Available at: www.bvs.co.uk/index.asp (accessed 25 Nov 2008).

Eysenck HJ. Dimensions of personality. In: Blinkhorn S. *Introduction to Psychology, Psychology of the Person (Unit 4): dimensions of personality.* Milton Keynes: Open University; 1981.

Festinger L. Cognitive dissonance. *Sci Am.* 1962; **207**: 93–102.

Freud S. New introductory lectures on psychoanalysis. In: Slack J. *Introduction to Psychology, Psychology of the Person (Unit 2): psychodynamics.* Milton Keynes: Open University; 1981.

Hamm RM. Clinical Intuition and Clinical Analysis: expertise and the cognitive continuum. In: Dowie J, Elstein A, editors. *Professional Judgment: a reader in clinical decision making.* Cambridge: Cambridge University Press; 1996. pp. 78–105.

Howlett E. *MRSA in London.* Health and Public Services Committee; 2005. Available at: www.london.gov.uk/assembly/reports/health/mrsa.pdf (accessed 25 Nov 2008).

Huffman K, Vernoy M, Vernoy J. *Psychology in Action.* 5th ed. Chichester: John Wiley; 2000.

Lister S. Patients beware that consultant with a tie to die for. *The Times.* 25 May 2004.

Miller F, Healy J, Toh T, *et al.* Doctor's pens: a potential source of cross infection. *Aust NZ J Surg.* 2003; **73**(Suppl. 1): A41.

Morrison V, Bennett P. *An Introduction to Health Psychology.* Harlow: Pearson Education; 2006.

Ogden J. *Health Psychology: a textbook.* 4th ed. Maidenhead: Open University Press/ McGraw-Hill; 2007.

Potter P, Perry A. *Fundamentals of Nursing.* 5th ed. London: Mosby; 2001.

Reason J. *Human Error.* Cambridge: Cambridge University Press; 1998.

Roper N, Logan W, Tierney A. *The Roper-Logan-Tierney Model of Nursing: based on activities of living.* London: Churchill Livingstone; 2000.

Roth I, Frisby J. *Perception and Representation: a cognitive approach.* Milton Keynes: Open University Press; 1992.

Salmon P. *Psychology of Medicine and Surgery: a guide for psychologists, counsellors, nurses and doctors.* Chichester: John Wiley; 2000.

Stuttaford T. Bow-ties are not the hygienic answer, so let's wash our hands of the matter. *The Times.* 25 May 2004.

Wallston K, Wallston B. Who is responsible for your health?: the construct of health locus of control. In: Sanders G, Suls J, editors. *Social Psychology of Health and Illness.* Hillsdale: Erlbaum; 1982.

Wilkinson R, Caulfield H. *The Human Rights Act: a practical guide for nurses.* Chichester: John Wiley; 2001.

CHAPTER 6

The interrelated nature of a psychosocial approach

In Chapter 5, I introduced you to a number of psychosocial theories and approaches in isolation, which impact upon the infection control behaviour of health and social care professionals. However, adopting such an isolationist perspective does not provide a true reflection of the interrelated way in which these theories and approaches impact upon an individual to influence their infection-control behaviour. Therefore, this chapter will present ways in which these theories and approaches act in a unified way to influence infection-control behaviour and the adoption of standard precautions.

I will begin by stating that non-adherence to standard precautions is psychosocial in nature. In part, such non-adherence can be explained through Freud's (cited in Slack 1981) structure of personality theory (*see* Figure 6.1) which will be applied throughout this chapter as a central theme with which other theories and approaches (*see* Figure 6.2) interact to cause non-adherence to standard precautions.

Figure 6.1 is intended to present causal reasons for both adherence and non-adherence to standard precautions through id or superego processes. However, in consideration of these two processes, human nature is such that individuals will always have the propensity to adopt an id-based process and will justify this by generating rationalised excuses (*see* Explanation box 6.1). This is because taking this route requires less cognitive effort (*see* Explanation box 6.2) than adopting a superego process (*see* Figure 6.1).

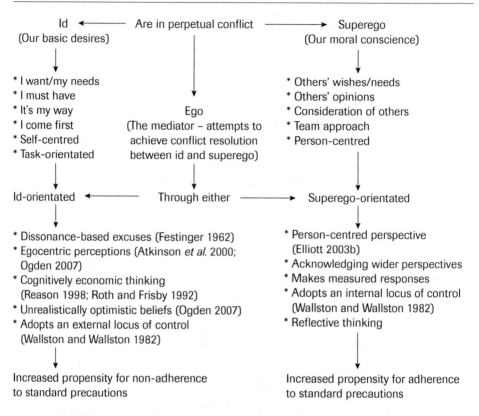

Id ⟵——— Are in perpetual conflict ———⟶ Superego
(Our basic desires)   (Our moral conscience)

* I want/my needs
* I must have
* It's my way
* I come first
* Self-centred
* Task-orientated

Ego
(The mediator – attempts to
achieve conflict resolution
between id and superego)

* Others' wishes/needs
* Others' opinions
* Consideration of others
* Team approach
* Person-centred

Id-orientated ⟵——— Through either ———⟶ Superego-orientated

* Dissonance-based excuses (Festinger 1962)
* Egocentric perceptions (Atkinson *et al.* 2000; Ogden 2007)
* Cognitively economic thinking (Reason 1998; Roth and Frisby 1992)
* Unrealistically optimistic beliefs (Ogden 2007)
* Adopts an external locus of control (Wallston and Wallston 1982)

* Person-centred perspective (Elliott 2003b)
* Acknowledging wider perspectives
* Makes measured responses
* Adopts an internal locus of control (Wallston and Wallston 1982)
* Reflective thinking

Increased propensity for non-adherence to standard precautions

Increased propensity for adherence to standard precautions

FIGURE 6.1 Linking Freud's structure of personality theory to multiple psychosocial factors.

EXPLANATION BOX 6.1 COGNITIVE DISSONANCE (FESTINGER 1962)

The concept of cognitive dissonance was originally identified by Festinger (1962), where he proposed that, at a psychological level, the individual will strive to make consistent two or more things that would not naturally be so. In simple terms, dissonance effects are when an individual generates excuses to justify their previous behaviour or behaviour they wish or intend to carry out. Hand hygiene is a good example, where the individual understands its importance in reducing cross infection, yet fails to adequately follow the hand hygiene process. Thus the individual experiences conflict between knowing what they should do and what they actually do or want to do.

Such conflict would manifest as stress in the individual and in an attempt to reduce such stress the individual will generate an excuse or reason for failing to follow the hand hygiene process. Such an excuse may be blamed on time, work load or an irrational belief that meeting other's needs must take priority.

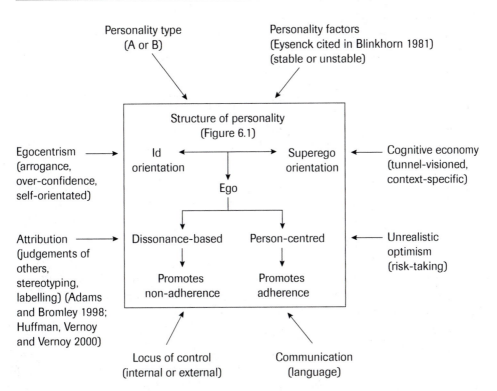

FIGURE 6.2 A unified approach to the impact of psychosocial factors.

EXPLANATION BOX 6.2 COGNITIVE ECONOMY
(ROTH AND FRISBY 1992)

Cognitive economy is where an individual has become context-specific or tunnel-visioned in their perception of what is occurring around them and will fail to take into account the wider implications of their behaviour. For example, instead of being patient-centred, the individual will become task-orientated towards achieving a set of goals that will meet their own needs at the expense of everything else and the needs of others.

Example: In the case of standard precautions, the individual will be context-specific towards achieving their allocated work load and as a result of this may:

- fail to change their gloves between interventions;
- fail to undertake or to fully follow the hand hygiene process;
- fail to ensure that they have removed all the equipment they used following completion of a procedure.

Adopting a superego route requires consideration of others and their needs, and therefore involves greater cognitive effort on the part of the individual. For example, most health and social care professionals will purport to be person-, patient- or woman-centred depending upon their profession or role in the way they interact with patients and clients and will believe as a result of cognitively economic and dissonanced-based thinking that their inter-actions and interventions are appropriate. Yet in primarily functioning at an id level, the individual will be orientated towards meeting their own needs over and above the needs of patients or clients. Therefore, the potential for the individual being task-orientated will be high, irrespective of what they may believe, because without being aware of it their thinking will be as economic as possible in an attempt to find the shortest and quickest route towards achieving their goals or needs. Such cognitively economic thinking and task-orientation will significantly increase the risk of non-adherence to standard precautions occuring. An individual whose thinking is cognitively economic (*see* Explanation box 6.2) will also have the propensity to experience unrealistic optimism (*see* Explanation box 6.3).

In reflecting upon this and current levels of non-adherence to standard precautions there can be no doubt health and social care professionals regularly take significant risks regarding their own and others' health and wellbeing. What is utterly astounding is that almost all healthcare workers, irrespective of their profession or role, know and understand the risks they are taking (West and Cohen 1997). Yet they continue failing to adhere to standard precautions. Subsequently cognitively economic thinking (*see* Explanation box 6.2) and unrealistic optimism (*see* Explanation box 6.3) are synonymous with risk-taking behaviours and beliefs (*see* List 6.1).

LIST 6.1 PSYCHOSOCIAL-BASED RISK-TAKING BELIEFS AND BEHAVIOURS

- the belief that wearing protective clothing (white coats, plastic aprons) will provide all-round protection for underlying clothing;
- the belief that if contamination of protective clothing cannot be visually observed then it does not exist and as such does not constitute a cross-infection risk;
- the belief that wearing work clothing to and from a place of work has no relevance to increasing the risk of cross infection;
- the belief that wearing a coat over work clothing when travelling home at the end of a shift will negate the risks of cross infection;

- the belief that there is no risk of cross infection when laundering work clothing with other personal items;
- the belief that laundering actually or potentially contaminated work clothing at 30 or 40 degrees Celsius will kill bacteria;
- the belief that failing to adopt standard precautions will have no adverse effects on themselves, but will have adverse effects upon others who fail to adopt standard precautions. This is closely linked to the 'It will not happen to me' syndrome (Elliott 2003a);
- the belief that the way an individual handles sharps or the containers into which they are placed following use will always be safe;
- the belief that because the individual does not make physical contact with others as a part of their role this negates the need for adopting standard precautions.

With regards to the risk-taking beliefs and behaviours outlined above you might want to reflect upon an experience I had many years ago whilst I was in clinical practice. On this particular occasion I saw an individual cleaning the inside lip of a sharps container with an alcohol wipe. In order to do this it required the individual to put their fingers inside the sharps container. A further example of a risk-taking behaviour which was relayed to me by my wife (who is a Community Nurse) and again involved a sharps container was when she saw a colleague deposit an empty vial into a sharps container. However, the colleague then realising they had failed to make a note of the batch number from the side of the vial proceeded to put their hand into the sharps container in an attempt to retrieve the vial.

EXPLANATION BOX 6.3 UNREALISTIC OPTIMISM (OGDEN 2007)

Unrealistic optimism is where a health or social care professional becomes unrealistically optimistic regarding the risky situation they place themselves and others in as a result of behaviour that constitutes unsafe infection control practice in the form of failing to undertake standard precautions or through failing to follow the hand hygiene process.

Unrealistic optimism can be facilitated through lack of personal experience. For example, a health or social care professional who has no or little prior experience of a patient's or client's health being directly influenced by their failure to adopt appropriate standard precautions will likely believe two things (Elliott 2003a):

1   There is no risk, or the risk of cross infecting others is so insignificant that it simply does not matter.

2 Even if there is a risk it will not happen to them. That is, even if the individual involved in healthcare does cross infect others, they will rationalise that is was not their fault (*see* Explanation box 6.1) or they will not be found out and held responsible and therefore, who cares?

Such economic thinking and unrealistically optimistic beliefs are heavily reinforced through the 'It will not happen to me' syndrome (Elliott 2003a). This syndrome is a defence mechanism against stress where individuals believe that an adverse experience resulting from dangerous behaviour will not happen to them and is reinforced by such unrealistically optimistic beliefs (*see* Explanation box 6.3) and dissonance-based excuses (*see* Explanation box 6.1), such as 'Because my clothing looks clean, it is. Therefore it is acceptable for me to go shopping in my work clothes at the end of my shift.' Yet such beliefs and excuses are rarely applied to others who carry out the same dangerous behaviour. In fact, individuals will readily apply criticism of others for undertaking the same dangerous behaviour they themselves undertake. In doing this, the health or social care professional will be able to psychologically transfer responsibility away from themselves for the dangerous behaviour they carry out. Furthermore, such transference will allow the individual to argue that because others carry out the same dangerous behaviour as they do, it must therefore be acceptable for them to follow suit.

REFLECTION EXERCISE 6.1

Can you think of situations related to the adoption of standard precautions where you have been critical of others for failures that you have been guilty of yourself?

If you have answered 'Yes', reflect upon why you did this and the ethics of your criticisms.

If you have answered 'No', reflect upon how you would feel about being criticised by a colleague for failing to carry out standard precautions, of which your colleague is also guilty.

Such transference is clearly irrational and is the result of dissonance-based thinking (*see* Explanation box 6.1) and unrealistically optimistic beliefs (*see* Explanation box 6.3). However, it will allow the individual to reduce any stress they might experience as a result of the psychological conflict created between the individual knowing what they actually did (*see* Figure 6.1: id process) and

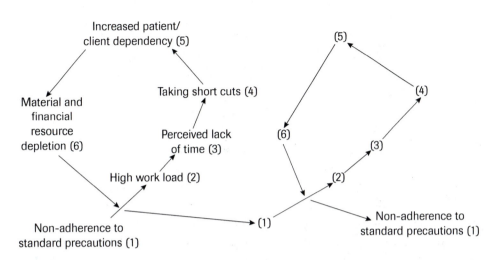

FIGURE 6.3 The standard precautions non-adherence spiral.

knowing what they should have done (*see* Figure 6.1: superego process). For example, the omission of standard precautions as a short cut to save time will lead to greater levels of work load, because failing to adopt standard precautions will lead to increased healthcare-acquired infections (Chalmers and Straub 2006). This, in turn, will lead to an increase in the length of time that patients and clients require health or social care intervention. Such short cut behaviour involving non-adherence to standard precautions is particularly prevalent when work loads are high. For example, where a health or social care professional has the unrealistic belief that because they have a high work load there is no time to adopt standard precautions. Clearly such a belief is rationalised (*see* Explanation box 6.1) and demonstrates cognitively economic thinking (*see* Explanation box 6.2). In this situation, what has been created for the health or social care professional is a psychological spiral (*see* Figure 6.3) where high work loads, perceived lack of time, taking short cuts, increased patient/client dependency and increased material and financial resource depletion will all reinforce each other in promoting continued non-adherence to standard precautions.

In this example, the individual knows they should not take short cuts where standard precautions are concerned because of the increased risks of cross infection. Yet they choose to do so as a result of following an id process (*see* Figure 6.1).

Before undertaking this exercise you might want to consider the following: time is an excuse we use to justify our failings. Yet although time flies you are the navigator and as such responsible for your time management (Elliott 1992).

In reflecting upon the above discussion, when have you taken short cuts whilst at work which could have increased the risk of cross infection?

Think about the excuses you used to justify taking these short cuts. Were these excuses rationalised as opposed to rational (Explanation box 6.1)?

We now have an individual who is highly susceptible to being self-centred, generates irrational excuses, is a cognitively economic thinker (*see* Explanation box 6.2) and a significant risk-taker – all of which can be linked to both attribution (stereotyping, labelling and judgements of others) and egocentrism (arrogance, over-confidence and self-opinionated) (*see* Figure 6.2). Egocentric individuals have a propensity to put their own needs first (*see* Figure 6.1: id process) and in placing their own needs first they are being arrogant and self-opinionated. For example, such an individual might say 'I am a qualified health professional and know what I am doing; therefore I cannot possibly be guilty of failing to adopt standard precautions!' Such a belief is a consequence of dissonance-based and cognitively economic thinking on the part of the individual. For the most part many health and social care professionals have such a cognitively economic and unrealistically optimistic approach regarding how they measure their undertaking of standard precautions against meeting the needs of patients and clients.

In reflecting upon this, I would argue that having to think about the consequences of failing to adopt standard precautions is a distinctly unpleasant activity and is perhaps even emotionally painful. Why? Firstly, because, as we have identified, it is always going to be easier to generate excuses and be cognitively economic and egocentric regarding our competence. A combination of these three will effectively allow an individual to be id-orientated (*see* Figure 6.1). Secondly, in being egocentric we like to consider that we not only know best, but that we also know what we are doing – both of which are assumptions many of us make. Yet such assumptions are highly questionable when linked with current levels of non-adherence to standard precautions and healthcare-acquired infection rates.

How egocentric are you?

Think about the answer you came up with and ask yourself: 'Just how rational is my answer?'

ATTRIBUTION

Although health and social care professionals profess to care about those they interact with as a part of their work-related or professional activities, many are only too willing to stereotype, label and make wholly subjective judgements about patients, clients and their colleagues, which are based upon highly questionable inferences (*see* Figure 6.2: attribution). These inferences are drawn from observing the behaviour of others, which is something identified within Chapter 5 as being highly questionable and extremely unreliable. However, it is interesting to note that health and social care professionals make these judgements with amazing consistency. Yet if the same consistency were applied to the adoption of standard precautions, it would surely result in a significant reduction in healthcare-acquired infection rates. So why do we make such attributions? Because in doing so it allows us to make sense of the world around us irrespective of whether such attributions are rational and professional. For example, using such labels as 'the schizophrenic', 'the single mother' or 'the homeless' can generate not only negative attributions, but also negative consequences in the way health or social care professionals behave towards such individuals.

Some examples of negative attributions are:

The schizophrenic:
➤ They should be locked up.
➤ They're all weird.
➤ Poor things – they're just retarded.
➤ Never mind – where there's no sense there's no feeling.

The single mother:
➤ Social services should be keeping an eye on her.
➤ I bet she's a drug addict.
➤ Look at the way she dresses; and she visits charity shops.
➤ I bet she was sleeping around when she got pregnant.

The homeless person:
➤ They must be on drugs.
➤ I bet they have fleas and smell.

> They're always in trouble with the Police for thieving.
> Be careful about touching them – you don't know what you will catch.

Some examples of negative consequences are:

The schizophrenic:
> Just remember, keep your distance or they will beat you up.
  The consequences to the patient or client will be isolation resulting from an irrational belief on the part of the health or social care professional.
> The mental health nurse who came with them can look after them.
  This kind of attitude on the part of the health or social care professional could result in harm to the patient or client because an assumption is being made that the mental health nurse has all the skills and knowledge necessary to care for them.
> There is no point in trying to talk to them as they will not understand what you are saying.
  For a health and social care professional to make such an assumption could lead to the patient or client failing to communicate important information regarding any changes in their state of health and wellbeing.
> Because they are mad they will not feel any pain.
  For a health or social care professional to make such a stereotypical assumption could lead to the patient or client experiencing pain when they need not have done so.

The single mother:
> There is no point in trying to hold a conversation with her as she is not very intelligent.
  For a health or social care professional to label the mother as not very intelligent is firstly reflective of an egocentric perspective, and secondly, could result in important information not being passed on by the mother.
> Be careful about getting to know her or the Police will be visiting you!
  For a health or social care professional to draw such a connection is both irrational and reflective of cognitively economic thinking, which could result in the mother feeling isolated and feel unable to seek help and advice. This, in turn, could have consequences for the health and wellbeing of the child.
> Make sure you keep your valuables safe or she may steal them.
  For a health or social care professional to adopt such a prejudiced perspective is making the attribution that being a single mother equates to them being a thief. The consequences of this for the mother could

result in anger at the healthcare system and a loss of self-esteem.

➤ I told her to pull herself together and she got upset! Make an entry in her notes that she is unstable.

This is clearly an unnecessary labelling of the mother based upon the health or social care professional's inability to communicate appropriately. The labelling of someone as unstable for being upset could have life-long consequences for both mother and child.

The homeless person:

➤ There is nothing wrong with them, they just want a bed for the night.

For a health or social care professional to be so cognitively economic in their thinking could result in them failing to recognise changes in the individual's state of health.

➤ Do not bother with an ECG, their chest pain is just gastritis.

For a health or social care professional to make such an assumption is reflective of economic thinking, which may result in serious harm occurring to the individual.

➤ No need to bother with standard precautions as there is nothing you could give them that they have not already had.

This is dissonance-based and cognitively economic thinking on the part of the health or social care professional because they are making the assumption that infection only travels in one direction.

The attributions individuals make allow them to apply cause or blame for a particular behaviour or social situation. For example, the doctor fails to wash their hands. In such a situation other healthcare workers might apply the attribution that all doctors are therefore responsible for cross infection. Such attributions are not only egocentric, cognitively economic, dissonance-based and unrealistically optimistic, but also must surely constitute outright hypocrisy – especially when considered within the context that in making these attributions health and social care professionals may be just as guilty of failing to wash their hands as those they are accusing.

REFLECTION EXERCISE 6.4

Upon reflection, is it possible that some of the judgements you have made about others' hand washing were hypocritical?

Consider this in relation to how well you have washed your hands in the past.

Such hypocrisy can be linked to the adoption of an external locus of control (*see* Explanation box 6.4) and an id process (*see* Figure 6.1).

EXPLANATION BOX 6.4 HEALTH LOCUS OF CONTROL (ADAMS AND BROMLEY 1998; WALLSTON AND WALLSTON 1982)

Locus of control consists of two dimensions:

1   Internal: This is the partnership between the patient or client and the healthcare worker, whether it is professional, administrative, managerial or ancillary. Such partnerships reflect the provision of information, non-judgemental attitudes and the right to ask questions without fear of ridicule and retribution. Such an approach is reflective of a biopsychosocial perspective.

Example: With regard to standard precautions, patients and clients have the right to have their questions answered in order for them to make informed choices as to whether they wish to comply with the advice given by healthcare workers.

2   External: This is where the patient or client is expected to be unquestioning, compliant and submissive to the demands of healthcare workers. Such an approach is reflective of a biomedical perspective.

Example: With regard to standard precautions, patients and clients are denied the opportunity to ensure that these are appropriately applied within the context of their healthcare experience.

The adoption of an external locus of control constitutes a failure to recognise and acknowledge the rights of patients/clients to be kept safe from infection, their right to life and their right not to experience torture (physical, psychological or social) and discrimination imposed by others. In addition, the adoption of an external locus of control would serve to negate an individual's right to security and freedom of expression (Wilkinson and Caulfield 2001). Yet the number of times health and social care professionals breach these rights through failing to adopt standard precautions is so high as to constitute sabotage (Parker and Lawton 2003). For example, the individual who seeks healthcare intervention and as a part of that intervention catches an infection that was not related to their original health problem, but was the result of a health or social care professional failing to adopt standard precautions, then such a failure must constitute an act of sabotage against the person.

The consequences of such an act of sabotage could impact upon a patient or client in such a way to have an effect on their right to life either through death or through the impact it has upon their future life span. For example, following catching the infection a patient or client may not be able to perform aspects of daily living (Roper, Logan and Tierney 2000) to the same degree that they were once able. Furthermore, where a patient or client catches an infection that was not connected to their original health problem, the principle of torture can be applied. For example, the experience of an infection may lead to patient or client suffering:

➤ physical pain from the effects the infection has upon their body;
➤ psychological pain from the emotional distress caused;
➤ social pain as a result of having to be isolated from regular human contact.

Whether it be physical, psychological or social pain experienced by the patient or client, if the infection was inflicted upon them by a health or social care professional as a result of non-adherence to standard precautions (because their employer failed to ensure that standard precautions were adequately undertaken by their employees) then that must surely constitute torture. Within this context, something that Florence Nightingale made reference to in her writings may be pertinent:

> I take leave to give the facts. We wait for the rates of mortality or injury to go up before we act and when enough have suffered we enter the results of our masterly activity in tables. But, we do not care to think about the consequences of our actions or omissions upon the patients or clients (Elliott 2003a).

This is a somewhat concerning perspective to which we might add that some 200 years later we continue to commit acts of sabotage against our patients and clients and inflict torturous experiences upon them through our failure to adopt standard precautions. Instead of acting in a person-centred way and following a superego process (*see* Figure 6.1) we choose to follow an id process (*see* Figure 6.1) where we hide behind our irrational excuses and our self-centred, egocentric (*see* Figure 6.2) attributions.

BREACHES OF SECURITY AND FREEDOM OF EXPRESSION

Every individual has the right to be protected from infection, yet, based upon current healthcare-acquired infection rates, adequate protection of our patients and clients leaves much to be desired. As for freedom of expression, although it may be appropriate to isolate an individual either in their own home or within a healthcare establishment, breaches of this right centre around two issues:

1 To what degree was the patient or client involved in the decision to isolate them?
2 Once isolated, the extent to which the patient or client becomes forgotten with regards to the meeting of their communication needs. For example, an individual who contracts an infection whilst in hospital and is moved to a single room or side ward. The door is then shut and the patient gets forgotten about, albeit unintentionally – an all too common occurrence. By being forgotten the patient's ability to communicate their needs whether they be physical (nutritional or elimination), psychological (emotional or afforded the opportunity to ask questions) or social (their desire for company or to feel included) is restricted and as such their right to freedom of expression has at best been impaired and at worst been denied. However, having read the above you might say the patient has a call button that they can press and that may be true. Yet, the point is that whether they have a call button or not the act of forgetting or omission is not a reasonable excuse ethically, professionally or in a claim for negligence of duty of care (Griffith and Tengnah 2008).

Infringement of these human rights and biopsychosocial needs falls within the context of an external locus of control (*see* Explanation box 6.4). In turn, the adoption of an external locus of control will be reinforced through cognitively economic (*see* Explanation box 6.2) and dissonance-based thinking (*see* Explanation box 6.1), as well as unrealistically optimistic beliefs related to the adequate protection of the patient or client's rights.

REFLECTION EXERCISE 6.5

In reflecting upon the above discussion, think about situations where, through non-adherence to standard precautions, you may have breached the human rights of patients or clients.

In contrast, the adoption of an internal locus of control (*see* Explanation box 6.4), where patients and clients are offered the opportunity to be involved to whatever degree they wish in their health or social care environment, will facilitate improved adherence to standard precautions. Allowing patients and clients to be involved in the management of their health or social care will provide a safeguard against non-adherence to standard precautions. This is because part of such a safeguard will allow patients and clients the option of offering challenges to the non-adherent behaviour of health and social care professionals. Offering such challenges will serve to raise the awareness of health and social care professionals to their dangerous practices. This will also serve to offset psychosocial factors (*see* Figure 6.2) and reduce the potential for following an id process (*see* Figure 6.1).

However, promoting the adoption of an internal locus of control as a safeguard measure against psychosocial factors (*see* Figure 6.2) presents three problems:

1 The human propensity towards adopting an external locus of control: doing so requires less cognitive effort (*see* Explanation box 6.2) than that required for the adoption of an internal locus of control.
2 Following an id process (*see* Figure 6.1): doing so will enhance the generation of dissonance-based excuses (*see* Explanation box 6.1) to justify adopting an external locus of control.
3 The potential for an individual to adopt a defensive posture when challenged: this results from egocentric and unrealistically optimistic beliefs (*see* Explanation box 6.3) related to the right of a patient or client to challenge them.

In contrast, the adoption of a superego process (*see* Figure 6.1) will serve to reduce the impact of such problems.

REFLECTION EXERCISE 6.6

1 Which do you adopt – an internal or external locus of control (*see* Explanation box 6.4) where your practice is concerned? Have you ever felt defensive when a patient or client has challenged or disagreed with you?
2 Make a list of when you have adopted internal and external approaches to the care of patients or clients.
3 With regards to standard precautions, was your adoption of them affected, depending upon whether you adopted an internal or external locus of control?

There can be no doubt that adopting an internal locus of control (*see* Explanation box 6.4) will always be a valuable factor in helping to safeguard patients or clients from the consequences of non-adherence to standard precautions. However, because of the powerful nature of the id process (*see* Figure 6.1) and psychosocial factors (*see* Figure 6.2) the propensity for an individual's behaviour to be controlled by them is extremely high. This is because individuals will always strive to promote the human need for

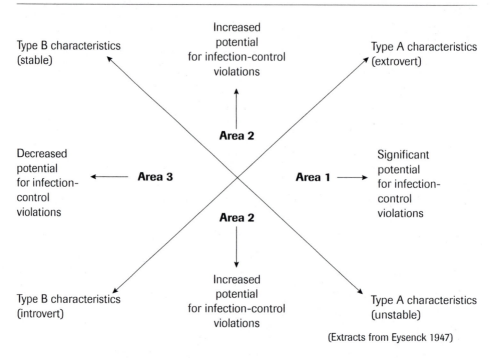

Type B characteristics (stable)

Increased potential for infection-control violations

Type A characteristics (extrovert)

Area 2

Decreased potential for infection-control violations

← Area 3

Area 1 →

Significant potential for infection-control violations

Area 2

Type B characteristics (introvert)

Increased potential for infection-control violations

Type A characteristics (unstable)

(Extracts from Eysenck 1947)

FIGURE 6.4 Extrapolating Eysenck's personality factors model and Type A/B personality characteristics to reflect the potential for infection control violations.

survival whether it be physical (safety from injury), psychological (safety from retribution or loss of self-esteem) or social (ostracised from a peer group). For example, the idea of continuing care where the work load is completed over a 24-hour period. In principle, the handing over of work load by individuals going off shift to those coming on shift should be a logical process. Yet for an individual the stress and anxiety that they may experience as a result of failing to complete what is perceived by both them and their colleagues as being their work load within a given time frame can be significant.

Such levels of stress and anxiety are generally underpinned by a fear of ridicule, retribution or social isolation by their colleagues. Sadly such ridicule, retribution or social exclusion is often the case where individuals fail to complete what their colleagues perceive to be their work load. As such, the need for psychological survival causes the individual to become cognitively economic in their thinking, resulting in them taking short cuts as a means of achieving the completion of their work load. The taking of short cuts includes failing to adopt standard precautions. Therefore, such short cuts serve to significantly increase the risk of harm that may occur to patients and clients. Adopting short cut behaviour can be linked to an individual's personality characteristics (*see* Figure 6.4).

Health and social care professionals presenting Type A unstable characteristics will be less reflective regarding the importance of adopting standard precautions. For example, the individual will be far less likely to adopt standard precautions if they are the type of person who needs to achieve more in less time because of perceived work load pressure and who is competitive and impatient regarding the rate at which a patient or client can carry out what the health or social care professional requires of them, has a tendency to underestimate when prioritising necessary interventions and is critical of others for the same acts of omission of which they themselves are guilty.

In contrast, the health or social care professional who presents Type B stable characteristics will have a greater awareness of their limitations, will be more effective critical thinkers, more able to pace themselves, more realistic in prioritising the patient or client needs and will be less time-orientated. As such they will have a greater propensity to adopt standard precautions.

PSYCHOSOCIAL FACTORS

Psychosocial factors reflected upon thus far (*see* Figure 6.2) will impact upon an individual's communication. For example, the term 'hand hygiene' (Elliott 2003a). However, in retrospect I feel it is necessary to acknowledge with regards to my previous publication that this term is only a partially correct description for a process of six stages (*see* List 6.2). Inherent within this process (Stage 4) there are three distinct methods – none of which simply involve the hands. This leaves the term 'hand hygiene' open to misinterpretation and assumptions regarding an individual's understanding of the term's precise meaning. Other terms applied to the same process are 'hand washing', 'hand disinfection' and 'hand decontamination'. However, as with hand hygiene, all of these constitute a dissonance-based, cognitively economic and unrealistically optimistic use of language related to a process (*see* List 6.2) that is far more than the sum of its parts. For example, the words 'washing', 'disinfection', 'decontamination' and 'cleansing' all have the potential to infer different meanings (*see* List 6.3).

LIST 6.2 HAND HYGIENE PROCESS (ELLIOTT 2003a)

Stage 1 – It is vital that you recognise the need to undertake hand hygiene. This is probably the most important stage within the process because if you fail to recognise situations where you need to adopt formal hand hygiene, as opposed to using cleansing gels, then the remainder of the process will at worst not occur and at best occur intermittently. Either way the risk of cross infection will be increased.

Stage 2 – It is important that you wet all areas to be washed thoroughly with running water. Failure do this may lead to you experiencing skin problems because some cleansing agents can cause irritation of the skin if applied prior to wetting the areas to be washed. The rule being always read the manufacturer's recommendations.

Stage 3 – It is important that you always apply an appropriate cleansing agent to the areas for washing. They type of agent will be determined by the nature of the intended intervention:
- invasive/surgical
- antiseptic
- social.

It is not necessary to apply excessive amounts of the cleansing solution and the manufacturer's recommendations should always be followed.

Stage 4 – It is important that you use running water when washing the areas of your body to be cleansed/decontaminated, using an approved method and time period:
- invasive/surgical: minimum 2 minutes – hands, wrists and up to the elbow;
- antiseptic: minimum 30 seconds – hands, wrists and up to mid-forearm;
- social: minimum 15 seconds – hands and wrists.

Stage 5 – It is important that you rinse all the areas washed, until all trace of the cleansing agent has gone. Failure to do this may lead to skin irritation resulting from traces of the cleansing agent being left on your skin. In addition, where traces of the cleansing agent are left on the skin this may serve to facilitate bacterial re-colonisation.

Stage 6 – It is important to thoroughly dry all of the areas washed, using:
- sterile hand towels for invasive/surgical interventions;
- sterile or disposable hand towels depending upon the nature of the intervention antiseptic to be used;
- disposable hand towels or hot air blowers for social interventions.

LIST 6.3 EXAMPLES OF WORD VARIATIONS

Here is a list of word variations and their meanings:
Washing:

- bathe, rinse, sponge down, wash down, sluice, swab, shampoo, launder

Cleansing:
- wash out, clean, flush out, sluice

Disinfection:
- sterilise, make germ-free, sanitise, fumigate, bleach, clean thoroughly

Decontamination:
- purify, clean up, neutralise, fumigate, cleanse

As can be seen from the content of List 6.3, although there are some similarities between the words there is by no means universal meaning between them. Taken within the context of the global society we live in, the potential for each of these words to be interpreted in a multitude of different ways is significant. This potential will serve to enhance the risk of non-adherence to this vital aspect of standard precautions. Furthermore, prefixing each of these words (*see* List 6.3) with the word 'hand' will again create the potential for misinterpretation regarding which of the three methods should be undertaken (*see* List 6.2, Stage 4). Irrespective of which word from List 6.3 is prefixed with 'hand' the propensity to cause an individual to infer that the hands are the only aspect of the upper limbs that are important for safe infection control practice is considerable. Subsequently, there is a need for a term that will encompass the upper limbs and not just the hands. As such, the phrase 'upper limb hygiene' would seem a far more valid and reliable title than any previously used.

REFLECTION EXERCISE 6.7

Reflecting upon the above discussion, can you think of a more universal term to replace hand hygiene, hand washing, hand cleansing, hand disinfection and hand decontamination?

CONCLUSION

In this chapter I have attempted to show how each of the psychosocial factors identified (*see* Figure 6.2) impact in a unified way upon an individual to affect the degree to which they will adhere to standard precautions. In reality, the achievement of consistent adherence to standard precautions among health and social care professionals is far more complex than is generally recognised.

REFERENCES

Adams B, Bromley B. *Psychology for Healthcare: key terms and concepts.* Basingstoke: Macmillan; 1998.

Atkinson RL, Atkinson RC, Smith E, *et al. Hilgard's Introduction to Psychology.* 13th ed. London: Harcourt College; 2000.

Chalmers C, Straub M. Standard principles for preventing and controlling infection. *Nurs Stand.* 2006; **20**(23): 57–65.

Elliott P. Accident and emergency training for nurses. *Mod Manag.* 1992; December issue.

Elliott P. Recognising the psychosocial issues involved in hand hygiene. *J R Soc Promo Health.* 2003a; **123**(2): 88–94.

Elliott P. Failing to adopt a patient-centred approach: a multi-professional problem, *BMJ* 2003b. Available at: www.bmj.com/cgi/eletters/326/7402/0#33297 (accessed 25 Nov 2008).

Eysenck HJ. *Dimensions of Personality.* London: Routledge and Kegan Paul; 1947.

Eysenck HJ. Dimensions of personality. In: Blinkhorn S. *Introduction to Psychology, Psychology of the Person (Unit 4): dimensions of personality.* Milton Keynes: Open University; 1981.

Festinger L. Cognitive dissonance. *Sci Am.* 1962; **207**: 93–102.

Freud S. New introductory lectures on psychoanalysis. In: Slack J. *Introduction to Psychology, Psychology of the Person (Unit 2): psychodynamics.* Milton Keynes: Open University; 1981.

Griffith R, Tengnah C. *Law and Professional Issues in Nursing.* Exeter: Learning Matters; 2008.

Huffman K, Vernoy M, Vernoy J. *Psychology in Action.* 5th ed. Chichester: John Wiley; 2000.

Ogden J. *Health Psychology: a textbook.* 4th ed. Maidenhead: Open University Press/ McGraw-Hill; 2007.

Parker D, Lawton R. Psychological contribution to the understanding of adverse events in healthcare. *Qual Saf Health Care.* 2003; **12**: 453–7.

Reason J. *Human Error.* Cambridge: Cambridge University Press; 1998.

Roper N, Logan W, Tierney A. *The Roper, Logan and Tierney Model of Nursing: based on activities of living.* London: Churchill Livingstone; 2000.

Roth I, Frisby J. *Perception and Representation: a cognitive approach.* Milton Keynes: Open University; 1992.

Wallston K, Wallston B. Who is responsible for your health?: the construct of health locus of control. In: Sanders G, Suls J, editors. *Social Psychology of Health and Illness.* Hillsdale: Erlbaum; 1982.

West K, Cohen M. Standard precautions: a new approach to reducing infection transmission in the hospital setting. *J Intraven Nurs.* 1997; **20**(65): 7–10.

Wilkinson R, Caulfield H. *The Human Rights Act: a practical guide for nurses.* Chichester: John Wiley; 2001.

SECTION 2

Moving towards consistent safe practice

INTRODUCTION

Within this section you will be introduced to the complexities of behaviour change (Chapter 7), several strategies that have the potential to positively counteract the psychosocial forces that were reflected upon within Section 1 (Chapters 8, 9, 10 and 11) and an examination of the controversial issues of challenging the status quo, and of public awareness and right to know (Chapters 12 and 13).

1   Chapter 7 sets out to reflect upon the complex psychosocial influences that make changing an individual's behaviour so difficult. The chapter proposes that behavioural change can be influenced not only by how an individual thinks (concept-driven inhibitors) but also by what they experience within their environment (data-driven inhibitors).

2   Chapter 8 offers a unique approach to facilitating adherence to safe infection-control practice through humour, play, interpersonal skills and music. Although the people who do this are referred to as 'clown doctors', this role can be applied to any health or social care setting and undertaken by any professional who has received appropriate training.

3   Chapter 9 considers the idea of reflection as a method of facilitating safe infection-control practice and offers an interesting approach to the idea of reflection.

4   Chapter 10 examines the process of clinical supervision and its potential to facilitate safe infection-control practice. The discussion sets out to define and redefine the term 'clinical supervision' and to reflect upon psychosocial theories and approaches that will influence the effectiveness of that clinical supervision. The discussion concludes by reflecting upon the idea of person-centred development as an alternative to clinical supervision and a strategy for enhancing safe infection-control practice.

5   Chapter 11 examines the potential for education to facilitate safe infection-control practice.

6   Chapter 12 considers the necessity of challenging the status quo in an open and frank manner, irrespective of whether or not individuals feel uncomfortable or ill at ease in undertaking such challenging. Many health and social care workers feel uneasy with the idea of openly challenging the status quo for fear of the reaction of colleagues or employers.

7   Chapter 13 examines the importance of raising public awareness to the dangers they place themselves at as a result of the unsafe infection-control practices of many health and social care professionals.

CHAPTER 7

The complexities of behavioural change

In writing this chapter, my intention is to introduce you to the complexities and difficulties regarding behavioural change and the fact that if adherence to safe infection-control practice is to be improved on a consistent basis then, in reality, behavioural change is what must be achieved. Throughout the chapter I shall discuss behavioural change within the context of adopting standard precautions. I shall also introduce you to broad areas that can inhibit behavioural change, referred to as 'concept-driven inhibitors' and 'data-driven inhibitors' (*see* Explanation boxes 7.1 and 7.2; Figure 7.1).

EXPLANATION BOX 7.1 CONCEPT-DRIVEN BEHAVIOURAL INHIBITORS

The idea behind the use of the term 'concept-driven' derives from psychology and may also be referred to as 'top down' (Pickering 1981). Both terms are intended to indicate that an individual's judgement and behaviour are influenced by neural activity or past experience within the brain or mind.* For example:

1. An individual's interpretation of audit tools and prescriptive rules may be influenced by the past experience of such. Were they user friendly?
2. Interpretation of another's behaviour is the result of their knowledge of a given person and their subsequent expectations.

---

* I have chosen to use the terms 'brain' and 'mind' because they both seem to be appropriate depending upon an individual's perspective. The term 'brain' might be used by a health or social care professional who adopts a biomedical approach and bases their understanding of the human body on a physiological perspective or perceives human behaviour as being caused by a series of chemical reactions within neural pathways. In contrast, the term 'mind' might be used by a health or social care professional who adopts a biopsychosocial approach and bases their understanding of the human body from a spiritual perspective or perceives human behaviour as being influenced by the soul and conscious awareness.

3 When others communicate with us, whether it is through verbal, non-verbal communication or the written word, it will be interpreted according to whether or not we consider what is being communicated to be true and whether or not the content of the communication is consistent with our attitudes and beliefs.

However, in each of these examples, such processes as cognitive dissonance, cognitive economy and unrealistic optimism will all have a major impact in determining whether behavioural change occurs or whether an individual's current behaviour is reinforced. With regards to these processes they are all determinants of the way each of us thinks and the beliefs we hold. As such, the idea of concept-driven is perhaps far more than a physiologically driven set of chemical reactions.

EXPLANATION BOX 7.2 DATA-DRIVEN BEHAVIOURAL INHIBITORS

The idea underlying use of the term 'data-driven' derives from psychology and may also be referred to as 'bottom up' (Pickering 1981). Both terms are intended to indicate that an individual's judgements and behaviour are influenced by information received from environmental sources through their five senses. For example:
1 Audit tools and prescriptive rules are physical entities that exist within the environment.
2 Interpretation of another's behaviour is the result of us observing them within the environment.
3 When others communicate with us, whether it be verbal, non-verbal communication or by the written word, they are all sources of information that exist within our environment.

Thus anything that is data-driven or bottom up emanates from the environment around us.

There is no doubt that achieving consistent adherence to standard precautions among health and social care professionals is at best difficult, and at worst impossible (Rollnick, Mason and Butler 2000). But why should this be the case? Why is it that health and social care professionals cannot simply be asked to change from a generalised non-adherence to standard precautions to adopting them in a consistent way?

Can you think of reasons why simply asking people to change their behaviour will not work?

In considering this, you might want to think about occasions when you may not have been willing to change the way you behave. Think about something you do that you know is bad for you or could cause you harm and yet you continue to carry out the particular behaviour. What would it take to make you change or stop what you do?

Identifying why people do not change their behaviour is related to the way they think and can be individualised, group- or society-based.

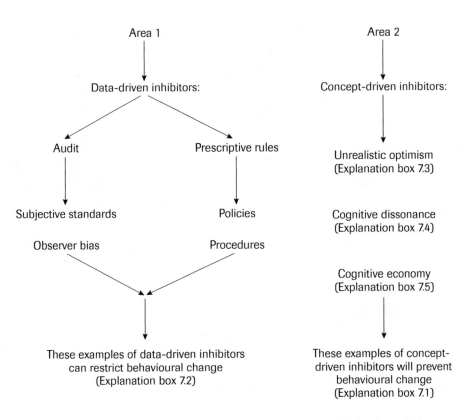

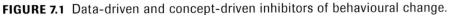

FIGURE 7.1 Data-driven and concept-driven inhibitors of behavioural change.

Individualised

The way a health or social care professional thinks about hand hygiene can be influenced by the attitudes and behaviour of their parents. As the primary care givers, parents will significantly influence the behaviour of their children. From the child's perspective, copying their parents can be both nature- and nurture-related. The child will learn through social experiences (nurture); for example, when and why to wash hands. However, the child will also learn to copy their parents' behaviour through the action of mirror neurons (nature) (Dobbs 2006), which provide each of us with an innate ability to copy others' behaviour. Both social experience and mirror neurons are in themselves powerful forces and when combined they will become primary determinants of behaviour (Plowman 2006).

Group-based influence

Peer groups can influence a health or social care professional's thinking about the adoption of standard precautions. By their nature, humans are social animals and as such have a basic need to feel included (Corsano, Majorano and Champretavy 2006). Therefore, individuals will have the propensity to align or role model themselves with the behaviour of their peers or those they perceive to be powerful. However, this propensity will not simply be the result of social experience (nurture), but will be the continued influence of mirror neurons (nature) (Dobbs 2006). Furthermore, the influence these mirror neurons have upon an individual's ability to copy the behaviour of others will be enhanced if the individual perceives those others as holding authority or as being knowledgeable. Thus the combination of nature and nurture will continue to be a powerful determinant of an individual's behaviour (Plowman 2006) following entry to the health professions and receiving education and training in safe infection-control practice. However, inconsistency between what a health or social care professional has learnt from their parents and what they observe in the behaviour of their peer group can lead to psychological conflict. Such conflict will, in turn, cause the individual to experience stress. In such a situation, concept-driven inhibitors (*see* Figure 7.1; Explanation box 7.1) will begin to exert an influence over how the health or social care professional resolves the conflict and their stress. In essence what the individual will do is attempt to find similarities between what they have learnt from their parents and the behaviour of their colleagues. In determining such similarities, the individual will then be able to reduce their stress. Furthermore, these similarities will be reinforced by concept-driven inhibitors (*see* Figure 7.1; Explanation boxes 7.1, 7.3, 7.4 and 7.5).

EXPLANATION BOX 7.3 UNREALISTIC OPTIMISM (OGDEN 2007)

Unrealistic optimism is where a health or social care professional becomes unrealistically optimistic regarding the risky situation they place themselves and others in as a result of behaviour that constitutes unsafe infection control practice in the form of failing to undertake standard precautions or through failing to follow the hand hygiene process.

Unrealistic optimism can be facilitated through lack of personal experience. For example, a health or social care professional who has no prior experience of a patient's or client's health being directly influenced by their failure to adopt appropriate standard precautions will likely believe two things (Elliott 2003):

1 There is no risk, or the risk of cross infecting others is so insignificant that it simply does not matter.
2 Even if there is a risk it will not happen to them. That is, even if the individual involved in healthcare does cross infect others they will rationalise that it was not their fault (*see* Explanation box 7.4) or they will not be found out and held responsible and therefore, who cares?

EXPLANATION BOX 7.4 COGNITIVE DISSONANCE (FESTINGER 1962)

The concept of cognitive dissonance was originally identified by Festinger (1962), where he proposed that, at a psychological level, the individual will strive to make consistent two or more things that would not naturally be so. In simple terms, dissonance effects are when an individual generates excuses to justify their previous behaviour or behaviour they wish or intend to carry out. Hand hygiene is a good example, where the individual understands its importance in reducing cross infection, yet fails to adequately follow the hand hygiene process. Thus the individual experiences conflict between knowing what they should do and what they actually do or want to do.

Such conflict would manifest as stress in the individual and in an attempt to reduce such stress the individual will generate an excuse or reason for failing to follow the hand hygiene process. Such an excuse may be blamed on time, work load or an irrational belief that meeting other's needs must take priority.

EXPLANATION BOX 7.5 COGNITIVE ECONOMY
(ROTH AND FRISBY 1992)

Cognitive economy is where an individual has become context-specific or tunnel-visioned in their perception of what is occurring around them and will fail to take into account the wider implications of their behaviour. For example, instead of being patient-centred, the individual will become task-orientated towards achieving a set of goals that will meet their own needs at the expense of everything else and the needs of others.

Example: In the case of standard precautions, the individual will be context-specific towards achieving their allocated work load and as a result of this may:

- fail to change their gloves between interventions;
- fail to undertake or to fully follow the hand hygiene process;
- fail to ensure that they have removed all the equipment they used following completion of a procedure.

Society-based influence

Using the example of drying the hands after washing, social pressures to behave in particular ways are often present; for example, sometimes there is a queue of individuals who have washed their hands and are waiting to use a hot air dryer. In this situation, the individual drying their hands can feel pressured into not ensuring that their hands are properly dry before moving off. As with individualised and peer influences, such social pressure can be a powerful determinant of behaviour (Plowman 2006). However, such social pressures can also be reinforced by the action of mirror neurons (Dobbs 2006). For example, if an individual waiting in a queue to dry their hands observes another person failing to dry their hands effectively as a result of social pressure, it may be that they will intuitively copy that individual's behaviour. This is because they will not want to experience the same social pressures and will justify failing to dry their hands appropriately through the application of concept-driven inhibitors (*see* Figure 7.1; Explanation boxes 7.1, 7.3, 7.4 and 7.5).

In reflecting upon these inhibitors (*see* Figure 7.1; Explanation boxes 7.1 and 7.2) let's begin by focusing on two data-driven examples: audit and pre-scriptive rules. Currently, clinical and educational audits are used within the context of infection control to identify areas of adherence/non-adherence and to provide a catalyst for improving adherence to standard precautions among health and social care professionals. However, the success of such

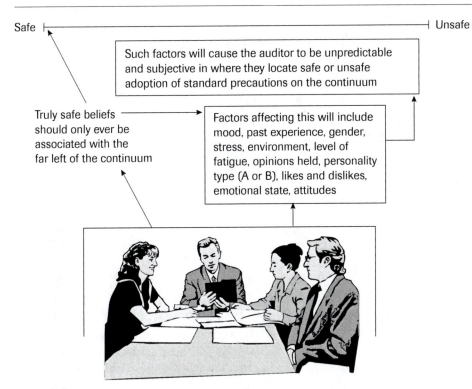

Safe ├───┤ Unsafe

Such factors will cause the auditor to be unpredictable and subjective in where they locate safe or unsafe adoption of standard precautions on the continuum

Truly safe beliefs should only ever be associated with the far left of the continuum

Factors affecting this will include mood, past experience, gender, stress, environment, level of fatigue, opinions held, personality type (A or B), likes and dislikes, emotional state, attitudes

FIGURE 7.2 Beliefs about safe and unsafe standard precautions: a continuum.

TABLE 7.1 Auditor's thinking/practice continuum

Levels	Definition
Level 1: Research-based thinking	Auditor supports their judgement with published research
Level 2: Evidence-based thinking	Auditor supports their judgement with clinical evidence
Level 3: Reflective thinking	Auditor supports their judgement in or on action reflection
Level 4: System-supported thinking	Auditor supports their judgement with information provided by previous audits
Level 5: Peer-generated thinking	Auditor supports their judgement based upon what others say to them
Level 6: Intuitive thinking	Auditor supports their judgement based upon their own subjective feelings, emotions and past experiences

(Adapted from Hamm cited in Dowie and Elstein 1996)

audits leading to behavioural change is questionable for several reasons. Firstly, the individual(s) completing the audit will determine what constitutes appropriate adoption of standard precautions according to their own subjective standards of safe and unsafe practice, even if they have a script to guide them. Unfortunately, such standards will vary between individuals and there is no universal demarcation of where safe practice becomes unsafe or vice versa (*see* Figure 7.2). Therefore, an auditor's judgement will primarily be based upon their subjective beliefs and will be the result of intuitive and/or peer-based thinking (*see* Table 7.1).

Safe practice will be facilitated if an individual's thinking reflects a flow between all levels of the above continuum. Various examples of the auditor's thinking/practice are outlined below:

Example 1: An auditor whose judgements are determined as a result of functioning at one level in isolation within the continuum (*see* Table 7.1) will be unsafe in their assessment of whether or not standard precautions have been appropriately adopted and applied. For example, judgements that are made on the basis of research evidence in isolation may be just as suspect as those made on intuition alone. This is because we should not necessarily believe everything we read simply because it

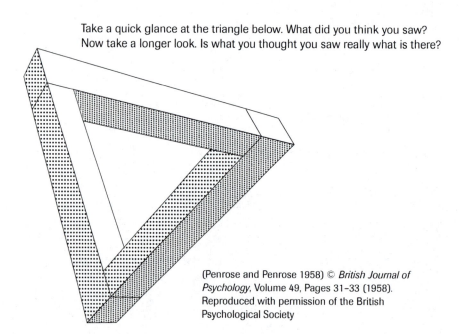

Take a quick glance at the triangle below. What did you think you saw? Now take a longer look. Is what you thought you saw really what is there?

(Penrose and Penrose 1958) © *British Journal of Psychology*, Volume 49, Pages 31–33 (1958). Reproduced with permission of the British Psychological Society

FIGURE 7.3 What you see and what is really there.

is in print and authored by apparently eminent or academically qualified individuals.

Example 2: An auditor whose judgements are formulated using all levels
of the continuum will be more likely to reflect the principle that truly
safe adoption of standard precautions can only exist at the safe end of
the safe/unsafe continuum (*see* Figure 7.2).

The fact that the auditor should have an audit tool to facilitate their judgements
will have little impact upon their determination of others' behaviour and the
subsequent judgements they make. This is because an individual's beliefs
about another's behaviour, which they will accept as being true, will have a
greater influence upon the judgements they make than what is presented to
them in the audit tool. In effect, the audit tool is a static entity that provides a
series of fixed statements that have been determined by others and which the
auditor may or may not agree with or for that matter understand. This is particularly so if they conflict with the auditor's beliefs. As such, these statements
may not be perceived by the auditor as constituting truths, which will lead to
them being rejected by the auditor. For the auditor, their beliefs will constitute
first-hand information, whereas that contained within the audit tool will be
second-hand information. Therefore, individuals will place greater reliance on
their beliefs, which to them are representative of what is true.

This indicates that what is recorded on the audit form will not necessarily
truly reflect the safe adoption of standard precautions. The reason for this
centres around what the auditor believes they have observed, which may not
have been what was actually being presented to them. In essence, the auditor
has seen what they expected to see (*see* Figure 7.3).

With regards to Figure 7.3 it is likely that at first glance what you thought
you saw was a triangle. However, having taken a closer look, is what you
see really a triangle? Your answer may have varied between 'Yes', 'No', 'Well,
maybe', 'Perhaps not'. In fact, the harder you look, the harder it may be for
you to make up your mind. Try and trace the outline of the object in the same
way you would trace around the outline of a true triangle. Are you able to do
this? Is there any part of the triangle that truly matches your perception of
what a triangle should be? In fact, this is known as an 'impossible structure'
(Pickering 1981).

I have used this object to highlight just how easy it is to fool our perception
of things. In effect, humans are not always very good at seeing what is in front
of them. In many cases, what we see will be heavily influenced by what we
want to see and what we expect to see. These wants and expectations can be
heavily influenced by dissonance effects, cognitive economy and unrealistic

optimism (*see* Explanation boxes 7.3, 7.4 and 7.5), which is why errors are the result of misperceptions.

A clinical example can be extrapolated from patient/client behaviour. Take the situation where an individual has a naturally loud voice. As far as this individual is concerned, they are speaking to you perfectly normally; however, you may interpret this loud voice as shouting, rudeness or possibly even aggression. You then go and make verbal and written reports of this event in which you record your perception of events. For example, 'He shouted at me in a verbally aggressive manner!' You then make you colleagues aware of your stereotypical and misperceived interpretation. As a result of your actions, you have now condemned this individual to being classified/labelled as something they are not – yet in reality you simply failed to take account of individual differences.

The object presented in Figure 7.3 is an example of how easily our perception and interpretation of what we observe can be fooled. It is therefore not surprising that many of the judgements we make are questionable. Observation is a principle method by which information is gathered when undertaking audits. This then presents us with observer bias from two perspectives. The first bias is that the auditor believes that what they are observing is a truthful interpretation of what is happening. Their interpretation of how well an individual undertakes, for example, hand hygiene, will have a greater propensity to be based upon the auditor's previous knowledge of that health or social care professional, whether they like or dislike the individual, that professional's status, the auditors pre-conceived expectations of how well or not the professional will undertake hand hygiene and the auditor's belief regarding what constitutes safe and unsafe practice (*see* Figure 7.2).

REFLECTION EXERCISE 7.2

What is truth? Is there any such thing as an absolute truth?

Think of something that you know and believe to be absolutely true and write it down.

Now ask yourself, how do I know this is true and can I prove it?

In reflecting upon this, there may be discrepancies between what you believe is truth and being able to prove it. For example, let's refer back to Figure 7.3 and the triangle exercise. When you first looked at this object you may have seen a triangle and believed your decision to be true. However, when you looked more closely it should have become apparent that the figure was not a true triangle at all. Therefore, this makes your original belief questionable as truth.

My point is that truth is something each of us decides about a person, place, object or observation. However, what we believe to be true does not make it so. In reality, I would suggest that there is no such thing as an absolute truth, except perhaps death, and even that can be questionable depending upon your spiritual beliefs.

In undertaking this exercise, I hope that you have begun to question the link between what we believe to be true and actual reality.

The second bias is that if the health or social care professional knows they are being audited on their hand hygiene they will almost certainly adapt their behaviour to match what they believe the auditor is looking for.

REFLECTION EXERCISE 7.3

Has there ever been an occasion when you were being observed that you changed your behaviour to what you felt matched what the observer was looking for? A visit to your working area by an Infection Control Specialist might be such an occasion.

Having reflected upon this, how great was the change in your behaviour from what you would normally do?

What the individual believes the auditor is looking for and what the auditor wishes to see may be quite different. In addition, once the auditor has departed, the individual will then almost certainly return to their original hand hygiene behaviour, which may or may not be consistent with safe practice. The observer bias here is related to the temporary behavioural change made by the individual in attempting to please the auditor and as such reduce the risk of any possible retribution. However, such temporary changes in behaviour can have serious consequences for patients' and clients' health and wellbeing. Yet the auditor accepts what they have observed the individual doing whilst undertaking hand hygiene to be a reflection of their usual practice and will have recorded this on the audit documentation. Such a record is then generally considered to be a permanent, valid and reliable notation of that professional's hand hygiene behaviour. Unfortunately, what is recorded may not be any of these.

For example, if the auditing individual is the manager of a given area and it is their area they are auditing then they will have a vested interest in demonstrating that appropriate hand hygiene is adopted within that area. As such this manager will have the propensity, albeit without any conscious awareness of what they are doing, to manipulate what they record on the audit documentation. This is a result of their interpretations being formulated out of what they wanted to observe happening or what they expected to happen as opposed to what was actually happening. In both of these examples, observer bias will act as an inhibitor to behavioural change. Therefore, the undertaking of an audit will be unlikely to lead to any consistent change of behaviour regarding the adoption of standard precautions by individuals involved in the provision of health and social care.

As such, when an individual is undertaking an audit of, for example the adoption of standard precautions or a single aspect of such they must ensure their awareness is raised to the potential fallibility of their observations and the inferences/conclusion they will subsequently draw.

Where prescriptive rules (policies or procedures) are concerned there is evidence to show that these have not been successful in effecting behavioural change (Lawton and Parker 1999, 2002; Reason, Parker and Lawton 1998) and it can certainly be argued that this is the case where the adoption of standard precautions is concerned.

REFLECTION EXERCISE 7.4

Why do you think health and social care professionals fail to comply with prescriptive rules that are supposed to enhance their safety?

Can you think of any reasons why the implementation of prescriptive rules will serve to inhibit health and social care professionals changing their behaviour to a more consistent adoption of standard precautions?

LIST 7.1 FACTORS THAT WILL INHIBIT BEHAVIOURAL CHANGE

Behavioural change will be inhibited by:
- being told you must change;
- the change conflicts with your attitudes and beliefs;
- the change conflicts with the opinions of your peer group;
- lack of consultation regarding the change;
- a perception that the change will have no gains for you ('What is in it for me?');
- not perceiving any need for a change;
- perceiving that not changing will have any consequences for you ('It will not happen to me' syndrome [Elliott 2003]);

- you perceive other priorities as having greater importance than any change;
- imposed change;
- stress and fatigue;
- where the change required is not explained;
- where not changing is reinforced by concept-driven processes (*see* Figure 7.1; Explanation box 7.1);
- where not changing is reinforced by data-driven processes (*see* Figure 7.1; Explanation box 7.2);
- authoritarian, dehumanising, condescending and egocentric styles of communication;
- no contact with the person or persons requiring you to change;
- lack of understanding of why the change is necessary;
- threats of retribution;
- having no choice;
- low morale, low self-esteem and apathy.

In addition to those presented within List 7.1, below are some indicators as to why prescriptive rules are poorly complied with and have failed in changing the behaviour of health and social care professionals:

1 Who develops these prescriptive rules and determines their content? Generally, where standard precautions are concerned it is infection control specialists. If compliance and consistent behavioural change is to occur, the development and content of such rules must be a team effort. That is, those who will have to comply with the rule, or a representative sample, should be consulted. If individuals do not feel they have been consulted and have some ownership then the potential for compliance and behavioural change will be poor.

2 How are these rules implemented? In general they are unconditionally imposed upon the individuals who will be expected to adhere to them. Imposing a rule upon an individual will always have the propensity for it to be ignored. Human nature is such that none of us like being told we must do something. Our human reaction is to reject what is being imposed upon us even if that rejection can negatively impact upon our health and wellbeing. For example, we know that non-adherence to standard precautions can lead to us contracting an infection. Yet, the level of non-adherence to standard precautions among health and social care professionals is staggering. The reason for such non-adherence could be related to the fact that we are constantly being told we must adhere to these rules. Imposing a rule on

an individual will not guarantee compliance with that rule or a change in behaviour leading to more consistent adherence to standard precautions (Reason, Parker and Lawton 1998, Lawton and Parker 1999).

3 Who determines language and style?

This is generally determined by the individual(s) writing the rule or by an employer. With any kind of rule that communicates via the written word, if the language used is not understandable by the target audience then it will be ignored and dismissed as worthless. In addition, the rule may be misunderstood and in its subsequent application in practice could result in harm occurring to the patient or client.

REFLECTION EXERCISE 7.5

Think about when you last read something you did not understand.
How far did you get through reading it?
What did you do with what you were reading?
What were your thoughts about what you had been reading?

In the same vein, if the style in which the rule is presented and formatted is not appealing to the eye, then again it will be viewed by the health or social care professional as being boring and will be dismissed.

REFLECTION EXERCISE 7.6

What makes you want to pick up a journal or book and look at it?
What influences your decision to do this?
In reflecting upon this, how often do you pick up a policy or procedure and read it? When did you last read your employer's policy/procedure for record keeping and infection control?

If a rule is to stand any chance of being complied with and effecting a consistent and positive change in behaviour, it must be user friendly and contain no jargon, no technical terminology that the target audience will not understand, and the language used must be universally understandable. As Winston Churchill is reputed to have identified, the United Kingdom and the United States of America are two nations separated by a common language. The same principle can be applied to the different professions in healthcare. For example, all professions arguably speak a common language but are separated by the jargon used by each profession.

4   What are the consequences to health and social care professionals for failing to comply with a prescriptive rule?

Usually the consequences are threats of retribution. However, compliance to a rule or as a means of achieving consistent behavioural change will never be accomplished through threats of retribution in the long term. To threaten something implies only the possibility of it happening. However, when such possible threats are measured against the 'It will not happen to me' syndrome (Elliott 2003) this syndrome will be successful every time. For example, as identified above within the discussion on audit, an individual may change their behaviour temporarily in the presence of an individual they perceive as holding authority. However, the moment that authority is no longer present the individual's behaviour will revert back to what it was originally because the threat is no longer present. Within this context, to threaten is a waste of time and the threat will not be considered as real until it is actually carried out. In addition, if a health or social care professional has no personal experience of, for example, someone being disciplined for non-adherence to standard precautions, then any threat of such will be perceived as fleeting.

5   What preparatory work has been undertaken to inform those who will be expected to comply with a rule?

At best the preparatory work is ad hoc; at worst, non-existent. Failing to keep individuals informed about a rule they will be expected to comply with will not enhance compliance or consistent and positive behavioural change. In addition, failing to inform could be considered a breach of the human rights of those who will have the rule imposed upon them within the context of the right to receive and impart appropriate information (Wilkinson and Caulfield 2001).

REFLECTION EXERCISE 7.7

If you are expected to comply with a rule, would you expect to be informed about the rule before it was imposed upon you?

Think about an occasion in the past when you were told, without any prior notice, that you had to comply with a rule. How did you feel about this and to what extent did you actually comply with that rule?

6 What time will be given to health or social care professionals to acquaint themselves with a rule?

At best the time is minimal; at worst, there is none given. Modern healthcare practice is a stressful experience and failing to provide health or social care professionals with time to assimilate prescriptive rules which they are expected to comply will:

➤ not promote consistent and positive behavioural change;

➤ not enhance compliance with the rule.

For example, from my own experience as a clinical practitioner within the National Health Service, I remember being presented with prescriptive rules, given a few moments to read them and then being told to sign a document stating that I had read, understood and would comply with the rule. Such expectations are clearly unrealistically optimistic (Explanation box 7.3) and cognitively economic (*see* Explanation box 7.5) on the part of those authorising such a practice in failing to recognise the potential consequences. They may also constitute a further breach of an individual's human rights within the context of prohibition of torture (Wilkinson and Caulfield 2001). As a result of forcing an individual to read, understand and sign to say they will comply with a rule without being given an adequate amount of time to assimilate the information, psychological distress and anxiety will likely be generated, as well as an increase in any levels of stress an individual is already experiencing. Those authorising such an action leading to psychological distress could be perceived as causing a torturous experience.

7 What has been done to inform health or social care professionals of the benefits to them in complying with the rule?

At best minimal information is given; at worst, nothing. Those responsible for developing prescriptive rules with the expectation that others will comply with them and make any behavioural changes necessary must recognise the necessity of presenting individuals with the benefits they will get from complying with the rule and changing their behaviour. This can be linked with Point 5 (above) in that failing to inform of any benefits could again be perceived as a breach of human rights in relation to receiving and imparting appropriate information (Wilkinson and Caulfield 2001).

8 How many prescriptive rules do health and social care professionals have imposed upon them?

There are an excessive number of rules imposed. Within their findings, Reason, Parker and Lawton (1998) and Lawton and Parker (1999,

2002) indicated that the more health and social care professionals are bombarded with prescriptive rules the more they will be likely to deviate away from complying with such rules. There is no doubt that the number of prescriptive rules that health and social care professionals have imposed upon them – and are then expected to comply with – is significant. Unfortunately, many prescriptive rules are imposed by management as a result of the potential for litigation as opposed to reflecting an altruistic approach to staff, patient or client welfare. My point is that if the rules are not being complied with they cannot benefit staff, patient or client welfare.

REFLECTION EXERCISE 7.8

How many prescriptive rules (policies, procedures or protocols) do you think you are expected to comply with? Try counting them up.

Why do you think many health or social care professionals fail to comply with the prescriptive rules they are presented with?

All eight examples given above will inhibit behavioural change because they are consistent with an external locus of control (*see* Explanation box 7.6). In addition, they will serve to deny individuals their rights of expression, individuality, choice, and their rights to give opinions and to receive information.

EXPLANATION BOX 7.6 HEALTH LOCUS OF CONTROL (ADAMS AND BROMLEY 1998; WALLSTON AND WALLSTON 1982)

Locus of control consists of two dimensions:

1. Internal: This is the partnership between the patient or client and the healthcare worker, whether it be professional, administrative, managerial or ancillary. Such partnerships reflect the provision of information, non-judgemental attitudes and the right to ask questions without fear of ridicule and retribution. Such an approach is reflective of a biopsychosocial perspective.
   Example: With regard to standard precautions, patients and clients have the right to have their questions answered in order for them to make informed choices as to whether they wish to comply with the advice given by healthcare workers.

2. External: This is where the patient or client is expected to be unquestioning, compliant and submissive to the demands of healthcare workers. Such an approach is reflective of a biomedical perspective.

Example: With regard to standard precautions, patients and clients are denied the opportunity to ensure that these are appropriately applied within the context of their healthcare experience.

With regard to data-driven inhibitors (*see* Explanation box 7.2), it must be recognised that the problems associated with achieving behavioural change do not lie with the idea of audits or prescriptive rules in themselves. Rather, the audits or prescriptive rules inhibit behavioural change because of the nature of their development, the human susceptibility to perceptual errors (*see* Figures 7.2 and 7.3; Table 7.1), the methods of implementation and the subliminal motives that sometimes lead to their use.

Moving on to concept-driven inhibitors (*see* Figure 7.1; Explanation box 7.1), within Chapters 5 and 6 it was identified that such processes as cognitive dissonance, cognitive economy and unrealistic optimism can impact upon our existing non-adherent and unsafe behaviour in allowing us to justify that behaviour. However, such inhibitors can also act to prevent behavioural change even though the individual may have some awareness that making the change being offered or identified is for their own benefit. For example, there is much published material that clearly identifies the importance of undertaking standard precautions (Elliott, Keeton and Holt 2005; Kermode and Jolley 2005; Infection A2Z 2005). Furthermore, within centres of higher education, despite the inconsistency between such centres being questionable (Elliott and Clark 2008), health and social care professionals are made aware of the importance of adopting standard precautions. Yet the influence these centres have had in improving non-adherence to standard precautions in the long term remains dubious. This is due to three factors:

1 The impact data-driven inhibitors can have upon effecting behavioural change (as discussed above).
2 The impact of concept-driven inhibitors. For example, dissonance-based excuses (*see* Explanation box 7.4) will allow the health or social care professional to establish what they believe are truthful reasons for not changing their behaviour. Thus the health or social care professional who argues that as a result of not making physical contact with their patients or clients the need to undertake appropriate hand hygiene does not apply to them. Such a rationalised, as opposed to rational, reason will directly serve to inhibit that individual from both recognising the errors inherent within their belief and changing their behaviour. Cognitive economy (*see* Explanation box 7.5) occurs, for example, when the health or social care professional has become fixated upon achieving a particular goal and their ability to see the

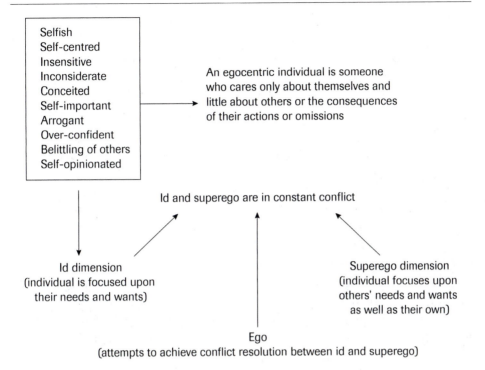

FIGURE 7.4 Defining egocentric.

need for behavioural change will have been inhibited. An example of this is where the health or social care professional needs to complete a clinic or ward round within a given time frame. In the past, as a means of achieving this goal they may have dismissed the need to adopt appropriate standard precautions when moving between patients or clients. This is because this strategy has worked in the past for the individual with no adverse consequences to them. As a result, they will become cognitively economic in their ability to recognise the dangerous consequences of their behaviour and will therefore fail to perceive the need to make any changes to their behaviour when undertaking a clinic or ward round.

3 With unrealistic optimism (*see* Explanation box 7.3), behavioural change will be inhibited as a result of the health or social care professional holding egocentric attitudes (*see* Figure 7.4) regarding their susceptibility to contracting, or risk of spreading, an infection through failing to adopt standard precautions appropriately.

Within the structure of Freud's personality theory (cited in Slack 1981) an egocentric individual would function within an id dimension. Such an individual would reflect the characteristics shown in Figure 7.4.

Such egocentric attitudes will serve to make the health or social care professional over-confident with regards to their risk-taking behaviour and any consequences to themselves. In being egocentric and over-confident the health or social care professional will inevitably become unrealistically optimistic about the consequences of their current level of adherence to standard precautions. Therefore the health or social care professional will fail to recognise not only the irrational nature of their beliefs but also any need to make any behavioural changes to the way in which they adopt standard precautions.

As outlined above, not only will the three examples of concept-driven inhibitors impact upon health and social care professionals independently, but they will also act in a unified way to inhibit behavioural change. For example, dissonance-based thinking resulting in irrational excuses to justify behaviour will be enhanced by such cognitively economic factors as a task-orientated approach to meeting patient or client needs and egocentric attitudes, such as 'I am the professional here and you are just the patient; therefore you do what I say!' Inevitably, each of these factors will inhibit behavioural change. However, when combined, they will exert very powerful psychosocial forces upon the individual to inhibit any behaviour change occurring and for the most part the health or social care professional will have no conscious awareness of the impact these forces are having on the way they adopt and apply standard precautions. For much of the time we are subservient to the influences psychosocial forces have upon the ways in which we behave.

CONCLUSION

In this chapter, I have attempted to enhance your understanding of the problems associated with behavioural change. There can be no doubt that getting an individual to change their behaviour will not be easy and therefore requires the identification of strategies that will serve not only to raise awareness of both the data-driven and concept-driven process involved, but also will serve to impact upon individuals in such a way as to enhance the potential for them to recognise the need to change their behaviour and then actually do so.

REFERENCES

Adams B, Bromley B. *Psychology for Healthcare: key terms and concepts.* Basingstoke: Macmillan; 1998.

Corsano P, Majorano M, Champretavy L. Psychological wellbeing in adolescence: the contribution of interpersonal relations and experience of being alone. *Adolescence.* 2006; **41**(162): 341–53.

Dobbs D. A revealing reflection. *Sci Am Mind.* 2006; **17**: 22–7.

Elliott P. Recognising the psychosocial issues involved in hand hygiene. *J R Soc Promo Health.* 2003; **123**(2): 88–94.

Elliott P, Clark S. *Report and Recommendations on Infection Prevention and Control Knowledge and Skills Acquisition for Pre-Registration Curriculum 2009.* Canterbury, UK: Department of Nursing and Applied Clinical Studies Canterbury Christ Church University; 2008.

Elliott S, Keeton A, Holt A. Medical students' knowledge of sharps injuries. *J Hosp Infect.* 2005; **60**(4): 374–7.

Festinger L. Cognitive dissonance. *Sci Am.* 1962; **207**: 93–102.

Freud S. New introductory lectures on psychoanalysis. In: Slack J. *Introduction to Psychology, Psychology of the Person (Unit 2): psychodynamics.* Milton Keynes: Open University; 1981.

Hamm RM. Clinical intuition and clinical analysis: expertise and the cognitive continuum. In: Dowie J, Elstein A. *Professional Judgment: a reader in clinical decision making.* Cambridge. Cambridge University Press; 1996. pp. 78–105.

Infection A2Z. *Standard Precautions.* 2005. Available at: www.healthcarea2z.org/stdPage.aspx/home/HealthcarePractices/HealthcarePracticesbackground/Standardprecautions (accessed 25 Nov 2008).

Kermode M, Jolly D. Compliance with universal/standard precautions among healthcare workers in rural north India. *Am J Infect Control.* 2005; **33**(1): 27–33.

Lawton R, Parker D. Procedures and the professional: the case of the British NHS. *Soc Sci Med.* 1999; **48**: 353–61.

Lawton R, Parker D. Judgments of the rule-related behaviour of healthcare professionals: an experimental study. *Brit J Health Psych.* 2002; **7**(3): 253–65.

Ogden J. *Health Psychology: a textbook.* 4th ed. Maidenhead: Open University/McGraw-Hill; 2007.

Penrose LS, Penrose R. Impossible objects: a special type of visual illusion. *Brit J Psychol.* 1958; **49**: 31–3.

Pickering J. *Perception (Unit 5), Psychological Processes: introduction to psychology.* Milton Keynes: Open University Press; 1981.

Plowman I. The four determinants of behaviour. *Proceedings of the APEN International Conference;* 2006, 3–6 Mar; Beechworth, VIC, Australia.

Reason J, Parker D, Lawton R. Organisational controls and safety: the varieties of rule-related behaviour. *J Occup Organ Psych.* 1998; **71**: 289–304.

Rollnick S, Mason P, Butler C. *Health Behaviour Change: a guide for practitioners.* London: Churchill Livingstone; 2000.

Roth I, Frisby J. *Perception and Representation: a cognitive approach.* Milton Keynes: Open University; 1992.

Wallston K, Wallston B. Who is responsible for your health?: the construct of health locus of control. In: Sanders G, Suls J, editors. *Social Psychology of Health and Illness.* Hillsdale: Erlbaum; 1982.

Wilkinson R, Caulfield H. *The Human Rights Act: a practical guide for nurses.* Chichester: John Wiley; 2001.

INTRODUCTION

I first met Bernie Warren some years ago at a conference in Oxford and whilst chatting to him I became very interested in the concept of clown-doctors and how such a concept could be applied to facilitate improved adherence to infection-control practice. Bernie is a Professor of Drama in Education and Community at the School of Dramatic Art, University of Windsor in Canada, and is the Director of the *Fools For Health* clown-doctor program and has considerable experience and expertise in applying the concept of clown-doctors within a multitude of clinical settings. Recently the Canadian Council on Health Services Accreditation, who accredits healthcare institutions nationwide, cited his *Fools For Health* clown-doctor program as a leading practice and recommended it as a 'standard for care' for long-term care (rehabilitation/continuing complex care).

I offer the following suggestions as you read Bernie's chapter:

1   Do not be misled by the word 'doctors'. Many of the principles employed by clown-doctors can be applied to any profession or role within healthcare.
2   You may wish to reflect upon how you could apply the concepts that underpin clown-doctors' practice within your working area as a means of promoting safe infection-control practice.

CHAPTER 8

'Hi Jean!': how clown-doctors help facilitate safe infection-control and positive healthcare practice[1]

Bernie Warren

SETTING THE SCENE: A BRIEF INTRODUCTION TO THE WORK OF CLOWNS AND CLOWN-DOCTORS IN HOSPITALS

Clowns have worked in hospital settings at least since the time of Hippocrates.[2] At the end of the 19th century, 'The Fratellini Brothers' (a famous clown trio) began the current tradition of clowns visiting hospitals.[3] Currently there are several models of practice for clowns working in hospitals[4] and presently clowns work across the life span[5] in hundreds of hospitals and healthcare settings in countries as diverse as Australia and Austria, Canada and China, Spain and South Africa.

The focus of this chapter is on the work of clown-doctors. However, much of what is described herein may equally be applied to the work of other professional clowns (whether they are called 'hospital clown', 'therapeutic clown', 'clini-clown' or simply 'clown'), whose focus is on healthcare, not just entertainment.

WHAT IS A CLOWN-DOCTOR?

> Doctors, nurses and other therapists work with the parts of the patient that are 'sick'; clown-doctors work with everything else.[6]

A clown-doctor is a specially trained professional artist who works in a therapeutic program within a hospital or other healthcare facility. Unlike clowns who make occasional visits to hospital bedsides to 'entertain', professional clown-doctors are skilled and valued members of a treatment team and thus an **integral** component of the healthcare process in the hospitals in which they work. Clown-doctors do not practise medicine in the conventional sense, rather (through the use of interpersonal skills, music, improvisational play and humour) they seek to help promote physical and mental health and to improve the quality of life for patients (or residents), their families and the healthcare staff who interact with them.

BEFORE WE BEGIN: TALKING WITH THE EXPERTS

Like most companies around the world, *Fools For Health* requires all prospective clown-doctors to undergo a full physical exam and makes sure that all employees' 'shots' (especially Tetanus) and TB status are up to date.[7] Moreover, prior to entering any hospital, clown-doctors are trained in basic hygiene and infection-control procedures – this part of their training often being delivered by the infection-control nurse.[8] In addition, all professional clown-doctors sign the same confidentiality agreements as their healthcare colleagues.

Prior to changing into costume and working with patients, clown-doctors get notes from, and ask questions of, their healthcare contact.[9] In chronic care wards or seniors' homes, this meeting may be comparatively short as the length of stay is relatively long and the clown-doctors can see an individual dozens of times. Usually this meeting focuses on any small changes in an individual's medical or psychosocial situation since the clown-doctor's last visit, with particular attention being given to any significant events that have occurred within the last 12 hours.

On an acute ward, where the clown-doctors may only see a patient once or twice, the information given can be very detailed. This meeting may take up to 45 minutes and may include information concerning the patient's medical condition and treatment as well as the pychosocial and family situation. Irrespective of the length of the meeting, information related to infection-control procedures and risks to both patients and clown-doctors are discussed. These may concern psychosocial and/or behavioural concerns (e.g. triggers for mood changes or violent behaviour), patients at risk from others (e.g. patients with neutropenia) and most importantly, precautions against such infectious agents as MRSA, respiratory syncytical virus, *C. difficile*, VRE or SARS.

TRIP AND FALL: HOW CLOWN-DOCTORS INTERPRET AND IMPLEMENT GOOD HYGIENE PRACTICES

On the wards and in residences, clown-doctors are advised to follow simple hygiene procedures. More than anything, correct hand washing and proper sterilisation procedures are emphasised! While each clown-doctor program is different, here are some fairly standard examples of hygiene rules:

➤ Do NOT come to work if you are coughing or sneezing!
➤ You cannot wash your hands too often. Wash with soap under warm water for as long as it takes you to sing the 'ABC Song'. If water and soap aren't available, use a hand sanitiser.
➤ **Always** wash hands at entry and exit from isolation and reverse isolation rooms and when leaving a ward.
➤ Do not put props bag on the bed.
➤ All props and instruments need to be cleaned thoroughly with soap and water or with alcohol swabs before and after visiting patients.
➤ Ideally, props should be cleaned between rooms, but always after they have been handled by a patient and **always at the end of the day**.
➤ When doing a clown-nose transplant, the nose belongs to the patient. There is to be NO sharing![10]

In practice things do not always go as planned:

> 'Dr Bigmon writes, "Dr Tilly and I were playing our tin whistles to an elderly patient when suddenly he grabbed my tin whistle and started playing. Then he gave it back to me and requested that I play another tune. As he had put his lips on the instrument, Dr Tilly and I made a big fuss about why we couldn't play our instruments anymore (something to the effect that he was too good, and now we were embarrassed to play after what he had shown us). After we left, we washed the instrument immediately so that we would not carry any germs to the other rooms we visited."'

By and large clown-doctors do not act as gatekeepers of infection control procedures. They do not make sure that individuals wash their hands or take their medications as prescribed. **However**, they do contribute (sometimes directly,[11] but more often indirectly) to controlling infections, promoting recovery from illness and speeding a patient's transition to good health.

It is, of course, very important that clown-doctors be seen to be setting high standards of hospital hygiene and cleanliness as they roam around the wards moving from room to room. Conspicuously using the 'hand santisers' and wherever possible making light of hand washing and singing the 'ABC song' is, of course, *'de rigueur'*! However, sometimes the *clown* gets the better of the *doctor*!

> 'Dr Foot-Twanger was keen to be clean before visiting a patient. He rolled up his sleeves, turned on the taps and started washing his hands. Soap and bubbles flowed. He washed everything: his elbows, chin, face, hat and, even his boomwackers! Dr Foot-Twanger became excited and thought he was under the shower so he started singing his favourite Italian opera with water and arms flying! He looked up into the room he was about to enter and saw the child cracking up and rolling around in giggles. Dr Foot-Twanger opened the door and all he could hear was "You're silly!".'

A LAUGH A DAY: PROMOTING GOOD HEALTH

Clown-doctors interact with patients, families and healthcare staff in hospital rooms and hallways, and visit patients and their families at their bedside. They talk with patients about themselves and their hospital stay. They play music and engage in short improvised stories and scenes – all of which serve to take the patient's and their family's mind off the pain and anxiety associated with their illness and generally being 'stuck' in a hospital.

Clown-doctor visits are usually non-threatening as they carry out no invasive procedures on the patient. Their painless visits leave behind smiles, often accompanied by a sense of wellbeing. As a result of the non-threatening and nurturing environment created by skilled professional clowns, most patients feel at ease and often talk freely about all aspects of their lives. Clown-doctors worldwide talk about how patients will share information that is unknown to other members of the healthcare team and **not** contained anywhere in patient records!

Often information is freely given to a clown that either puts the patient's behaviour in a new light or gives ideas about how to approach the patient or a family member. Sometimes this information is relatively innocuous, but every now and again clowns encounter information that is very valuable to the patient's treatment plan. The clowns can then share this information with other members of the healthcare team.[12]

> 'Recently, Dr Haven't-a-Clue and Dr Hoppy-go-Lucky visited a man they were told only spoke Italian, so the clown-doctors started singing a few verses of some Italian songs to him. The man, although wearing an oxygen mask, started singing operatic arias and while he was extremely sick he amazed everyone with the quality of his voice. Nobody else in his treatment team knew he could sing.

His singing aided his oxygen intake, helped strengthen his lungs and increased his lung capacity.'

I AM NOT SIMPLY MY DISEASE

'No one is ever dying.'[13]

Clown-doctors do not forget a patient's illness, but work with those parts of the individual that are healthy. They help remind family members and the healthcare team that a patient is not simply their illness. In doing this, the patient, their family and the healthcare team who are helping make them healthy again, are all able to see beyond the medical problem.

> 'Recently, Dr Haven't-a-Clue and Dr. Hoppy-go-Lucky visited a palliative patient once a week. They did not focus on his disease, but treated him as a vital human being. They sang and danced and joked with him and his wife, often talking about socially inappropriate and risqué topics. Nurses at the desk said that he talked about the clown-doctors during the week and looked forward to each visit. The attending physician told the clowns, "All I can do is give him drugs for pain; in many ways you are doing more for him than I can."
>
> For several weeks the clowns visited. At each visit everyone in the room knew that he did not have much longer to live, but for those few minutes when the clown-doctors were in the room he awoke from his stupor and was actively engaged and completely alive.
>
> On the last visit when the clown-doctors arrived at his room he was sleeping, but they were invited in by his wife and sang three soft songs. His wife thanked them for stopping by and they left. He died later that week. After he passed away the clowns received a note from his family: "THANKS a lot for everything. The clowns keep smiling for people that can't. God bless them."'

DIVERSIONAL THERAPY

Much of the time clown-doctors simply make institutions 'sparkle and shine', lightening the mood in hallways and rooms by smiling and joking. However, they also have to perform in difficult situations. As part of their training, clown-doctors have to learn to sing, dance and interact while wearing 'full metal jacket' (a gown, gloves and face mask). Sometimes what clown-doctors do is as much for the benefit of the parents or patient's family as it is for the patient:

'Dr BB and Dr Haven't-a-Clue were working on paediatrics on a day that the nurses were particularly stretched as the ward was full and there were many very sick young children to look after. On this day, the clown-doctors heard screams from down the hall. When they got there they saw it was an isolation room. The door was slightly ajar and there was a very young child screaming in her mother's arms. The mother and father were visibly distraught, so, while still outside the door, the clown-doctors began to put on their gowns, gloves and masks. All this time they were singing and dancing and smiling. Within a very short while the child was starting to smile. Before they had got all the necessary protective gear on, the child was smiling and giggling and clapping her hands in time to the music. The child had calmed down and the clown-doctors never even had to enter the room. More importantly, the parents were visibly relieved and the nurses did not have to be troubled.'

Much of what the clown-doctors do with children can be considered 'diversional therapy'[14] where they help to act as a distraction during minor bedside procedures; for example, while a nurse inserts or removes an intravenous drip, draws blood or gives an asthmatic a ventolin treatment. In addition, clown-doctors can sometimes find approaches to adult patients that encourage them to accept their treatment in a way that no one else can:

'Recently Dr Haven't-a-Clue and Dr Floretta Cauliflower heard an older woman screaming in another room. They quickly finished their work in the room they were in and made their way to the room from where the screams were emanating. On entering the room they found two elderly women. One was wearing an old fashioned oxygen mask over her mouth and nose, but she had been so agitated that the hose had come away from the mask. Dr Cauliflower held the patient's hand and talked soothingly with her. The clown-doctors started to sing quietly to her and slowly began to calm her down. While Dr Cauliflower held her hand, the clown-doctors re-inserted the tube into the mask. By the time the clown-doctors left they had engaged both patients in the room in various songs and everyone was smiling. Upon leaving, the clown-doctors went immediately to the nurse's station to report the incident and to ask if a nurse could go to check on the patient.'

CONCLUSION

In this relatively short chapter it is impossible to do justice to all the suggested benefits of humour and laughter in healing and illness prevention (Berk and Tan 1989; Dowling 2002; Fry 1992; Hudak *et al.* 1991; Mahony, Burroughs and Hieatt 2001; Martin 2001). Nor is it possible to fully cover all of the valuable contributions clown-doctors make to the healthcare process (Manic 2000; Oppenheim, Simonds and Heartmann 1997; Simonds 1998, 1999; Simonds and Warren 2001, 2004; Spitzer 2001; Van Blerkom 1995; Warren 2000, 2003, 2004a, 2004b; Warren and McAuslan 2002). However, our own research suggests that through the use of music, interactive dances and general playfulness, the clown-doctors help patients and their families:

➤ take their minds off the illness;
➤ brighten the mood of nurses, doctors and other healthcare staff;
➤ reduce anxiety in young children awaiting surgery (sometimes even accompanying them from the waiting room to the operating room);
➤ act as a distraction during minor bedside procedures;
➤ increase satisfaction with rehabilitation programs (based on various outcome surveys);
➤ reduce the need for pain and anti-depression medication;
➤ reduce the overall length of stay in the hospital;
➤ reduce staff absenteeism;
➤ extend the range of motion for stroke and aphasia patients;[15]
➤ encourage patients with a tracheostomy or aphasia to speak.

I will conclude with two quotes: the first from a unit manager and the second from a patient:

> 'Patients have commented that the clown-doctors made them work harder in therapy – almost in a competitive sense – and also that they allow them to have a bit of normality in their lives, for a few moments. When clown-doctors are near, smiles are everywhere. There is an infusion of endorphins into the air. Staff sing with them, react with them and, if needed, are quiet with them' (Bernice Markham, Nurse Manager, In-Patient Rehabilitation Unit, Letter to the Research Ethics Board, Windsor Regional Hospital, Canada).

> 'We should have the clowns here more often. I have a lot of fun with them. They bring sunshine and laughter. They put a smile on your face and it lasts the rest of the day and when you think of them [the clowns] it [the smile] comes back. They leave good feelings behind' (Stroke Patient (on Long Term Continuing Complex Care). Quote collected by Caroline Simonds **immediately** after Dr Twinkle-Toes and Dr Figzit had left a room, 17 June 2002).

REFERENCES

Berk LS, Tan SA. Eustress of mirthful laughter modifies natural killer cell activity. *Clin Res.* 1989; **37**: 115.

Dowling JS. Humour: a coping strategy for paediatric patients. *Paediatr Nurs.* 2002; **28**(2): 123–31.

Fry WF. The physiologic effects of humor, mirth and laughter. *JAMA.* 1992; **267**(13): 1857–8.

Hudak DA, Dale A, Hudak MA, *et al.* Effects of humorous stimuli and sense of humor on discomfort. *Psychol Rep.* 1991; **69**: 779–86.

Mahony DL, Burroughs WJ, Hieatt AC. The effects of laughter on discomfort thresholds: does expectation become reality? *J Gen Psychol.* 2001; **128**: 217–26.

Manic J. *Clownsprechstunde Lachen Ist Leben.* Bern: Verlag Hans Huber; 2000.

Martin RA. Humor, laughter, and physical health: methodological issues and research findings. *Psychol Bull.* 2001; **127**: 504–19.

Oppenheim D, Simonds C, Hartmann O. Clowning on children's wards. *Lancet.* 1997; **350**: 1838–40.

Simonds C. La douleur et le Rire, L'hôpital et le cirque, Les médecins et les clowns . . . Les enfants! In: *L'enfant et la douleur: familles et soignants.* Paris: Syros; 1998.

Simonds C. Clowning in hospitals is no joke. *BMJ.* 1999; **319**(7212): 792A.

Simonds C, Warren B. *Le Rire Medecin: le journal de Dr. Girafe.* Paris: Albin Michel; 2001.

Simonds C, Warren B. *The Clown Doctor Chronicles.* Amsterdam and New York: Rodopi; 2004.

Spitzer P. The clown doctors. *Aust Fam Physician.* 2001; **30**(1): 12–16.

Van Blerkom LM. Clown doctors: shaman healers of western medicine. *Med Anthropol Q.* 1995; 9: 462–75.

Warren B. Discovering connections between Eastern and Western approaches to promoting health. In: Turner F, Senior P, editors. *A Powerful Force For Good: culture, health and the arts – an anthology.* Manchester: Manchester Metropolitan University; 2000. pp. 60–2.

Warren B. Fools for health: introducing clown-doctors to Windsor hospitals. In: Warren B, editor. *Creating a Theatre in Your Classroom and Community.* North York: Captus University Publications; 2003. pp. 225–46.

Warren B. Treating wellness: how clown-doctors help to humanise healthcare and promote good health. In: Twohig P, Kalitzkus V, editors. *Making Sense of Health, Illness and Disease.* Vol 1. Amsterdam and New York: Rodopi; 2004a. pp. 201–16.

Warren B. Bring me sunshine: the effects of clown-doctors on the mood and attitudes of healthcare staff. In: Twohig P, editor. *Interdisciplinary Perspectives on Health, Illness and Disease.* Amsterdam and New York: Rodopi; 2004b. pp. 83–96.

Warren B, McAuslan P. What is the value of a smile?: an investigation of the role of clown-doctors working on an in-patient rehabilitation unit. 2002. (Unpublished conference paper.) For details of this paper the author of this chapter should be contacted directly.

NOTES

1 I wish to thank all the clown-doctors and therapeutic clowns around the world who have directly or indirectly contributed to this chapter. In particular, I wish to thank Caroline Simonds, Dr Peter Spitzer, Melissa Holland, Olivier Hughes-Terreault, Magdalena Schaumburger and all the clowns of *Fools For Health* for contributing more anecdotes and comments than could possibly be contained in such a short chapter. Wherever and whenever possible, individual contributors have been cited. The title for this chapter comes from conversation with Caroline Simonds about workshops she experienced in New York when working for Big Apple Circus Clown Care Unit.

2 As doctors of that era believed that mood influenced healing, Hippocrates' hospital on the Island of Kos supported constant troupes of players and clowns in the quadrangle.

3 While there were several precursors, 1986 is the date usually cited as the beginning of clowns working professionally in hospitals. In that year, Karen Ridd, a solo clown 'Robo' (also a child life specialist), initiated an experimental project at Winnipeg Children's Hospital in Canada. This became Winnipeg's Therapeutic Clown Program. At the same time, Michael Christensen (Dr Stubbs), along with Jeff Gordon ('Disorderly Gordon') first set foot in a hospital in New York. Their groundbreaking work led to the first clown-doctor program and to the formation of the Big Apple Circus Clown Care Unit. Both programs are alive and well. They have expanded and acted as catalysts for many programs around the world

4 For example, some clowns are also clergy ('Clowns for Christ'); others are simply 'entertainers' hired on an infrequent or regular basis; while still others are doctors who use humour as part of their medical practice. However, the two most prevalent professional ways of working are **therapeutic clowns** (aka hospital clowns) and **clown-doctors**. More often than not **therapeutic clowns** work solo while **clown-doctors** work in pairs.

5 Across the life span means working with patients of all ages, literally from cradle to grave. For example, the clown-doctors of *Fools For Health* see patients from as young as six days old (and their families) to as old as centenarians and all ages in between.

6 This quote is variously attributed to Ami Hattab (Dr Balthazaar), Kim Winslow (Dr Loon) and Caroline Simonds (Dr Giraffe) and most likely is an example of *Zeitgeist*.

7 They are also required to go through a background Police Clearance to make sure they have no criminal record.

8 The procedures described relate to *Fools For Health*. Other companies may have different procedures.

9 This is usually a charge nurse or patient care resource leader, or in the case of seniors' centres it may be a social worker or the recreation coordinator. The meeting is almost always done by the professional artist, 'inclownito' (i.e. before they change into their clown-doctor costume and assume that persona). In some facilities, clown-doctors receive a printed census or some form of short written history, which will include name and age of the patient as well as a brief medical diagnosis.

10 I am especially grateful to Dr Peter Spitzer (The Humour Foundation, Sydney, Australia) and Caroline Simonds (Le Rire Medecin, Paris, France) for their contributions here.

11 A good example of this is the early work of 'Robo' who often would help children learn to use their asthma puffers or walk with crutches.

12 Once again, all is conducted professionally, confidentially and in the best interests of the patient.

13 Attributed to Dr Hunter (Patch) Adams.

14 Carol Chism – tape-recorded field research.

15 Clown-doctors often work on the in-patient rehabilitation and complex continuing care units to help speech and language pathologists, physiotherapists and occupational therapists in their therapeutic goals.

INTRODUCTION

Janet Wiseman and I are colleagues within the Faculty of Health and Social Care at Canterbury Christ Church University, although we are based within different departments. I was particularly keen to have Janet write a chapter for this book to provide a social work/care perspective on infection control, which is an area where this topic is not always given the importance or attention it deserves. Janet offers a rather different perspective on infection control – one I hope you will find interesting.

CHAPTER 9

Reflection as a facilitator of safe professional practice

Janet Wiseman

This chapter seeks to draw attention to the importance of reflection in effective infection control. I will explore some of the barriers to reflection and how it can assist the development of good practice. Throughout the chapter I will present a number of reflection exercises aimed at drawing on the importance of reflection, and highlight misconceptions about reflection, gaps in knowledge and areas for development. However, although it is important for all those involved in healthcare and social work to apply reflection as a means of maintaining safe standards of infection-control practice, it is my intention to discuss the links between reflection and infection control within the context of social work.

Social workers pride themselves on their ability to assess complex situations and plan courses of action or intervention in an appropriate and timely way. To make these judgements they draw on the knowledge, skills and values acquired during the course of their education and training. However, it is also recognised that effective social work, which responds to the needs of diverse individuals in equally diverse contexts, requires more than the application of technical theory acquired during this training.

The use of reflection to increase or enhance knowledge, once the individual is in practice, can be a useful additional tool to draw on (D'Cruz *et al.* 2007). Its most useful application has been described as 'reflection in action' (Schön 1991), which can be applied to many challenging practice scenarios. Using reflection enables social workers to continue to build their knowledge and skills into a wealth of 'practice wisdom' (Saltiel 2003) and can be particularly useful when applying principles of ethical practice.

It can be argued that social workers have an ethical duty to be well-informed about infection control and to understand the implications of lack of knowledge in this area. However, social workers are unlikely to be fully informed about the issue and may instead be influenced by unreliable sources of evidence.

REFLECTION EXERCISE 9.1

Make a list of all of the words that come to mind when you think about healthcare-acquired infection.

What is it caused by?

Where has your current knowledge come from?

Pre-registration training
Workplace induction
Health and safety awareness training
Colleagues
Personal experience
Popular media.

For example, the popular media portrayal of the untoward spread of infection is that it is caused by unclean hospitals or poor hygiene procedures by doctors, nurses or domestic staff (Washer and Joffe 2006). It is also wrongly suggested by these reports that most infection occurs during in-patient admissions to hospitals. In this sense it might be easy for social workers to assume that they have no part to play in effective infection control. However, social workers certainly have a role to play and a responsibility to neither over- or under-react to the need for effective infection control. They need to use the established evidence base to become well-informed and, in particular, to understand that this is a core social work issue.

REFLECTION EXERCISE 9.2

Consider the list of standard precautions below (*see* List 9.1)

Reflect on your recent practice and decide which precautions have:
1 No relevance   }
2 Some relevance   } to you professional practice?
3 Significant relevance }

Then consider situations you have been in where standard precautions would have had some or significant relevance.

How well do you feel prepared to address these precautions?

LIST 9.1 STANDARD PRECAUTIONS

1 **Recognising the need** to adopt standard precautions is the most important aspect. Failing to recognise the need will be governed by the way an individual thinks, which will, in turn, impact upon their perception of the relevance and importance of such precautions. If an individual perceives standard precautions as being irrelevant, unimportant or of less priority, then the potential for non-adherence will be significantly increased.

2 **Hand hygiene** is vital in facilitating the prevention and reduction of healthcare-acquired infections. Hand hygiene must be carried out frequently, with individuals constantly reflecting upon the principle of, 'What have I just done and what am I going to do now?' If the *just done* constitutes a risk to themselves or others then appropriate hand hygiene must be undertaken prior to proceeding to the *do now*. Further, consideration must also be given to the full undertaking of the hand hygiene process.

3 **Hand rubs** are an effective method of hand decontamination in the short term. However, they should never be perceived as an absolute substitute for adoption of formal hand hygiene using the hand hygiene process.

4 **Disposable aprons** can provide some protection for the wearer. However, they should never be perceived as an absolute barrier and must be changed frequently. As a general rule the *just done, do now* approach should be adopted at all times.

5 **Disposable gloves** must always be worn when handling body fluids or any contaminated substance/materials. As a general rule, if in doubt wear gloves. Management and/or colleagues should not presume to ridicule or restrict an individual's decision to wear gloves.

6 **Skin trauma** must be dealt with in accordance with your employer's policies and procedures and in accordance with health and safety law. All trauma to the skin, irrespective of how minor, must be cleaned, dried, covered and reported. It is a legal requirement that an accident/incident form is completed and individuals should report to either the occupational health department or to accident and emergency.

7 **The eyes** should be protected where there is either a potential or actual risk of flying debris or splashes of body fluids/harmful substances. Individuals must determine for themselves when the wearing of appropriate eye

protection is necessary. Management should not presume to restrict such determinations or they may be in contravention of an individual's human rights.

8 **Sharps** are dangerous and will cause harm. A sharps injury may have consequences for the remainder of an individual's life span. A 'sharp' may be defined as anything that can either penetrate or cause trauma to the skin. Always handle sharps with caution whilst giving consideration to the safety of those around you. The rule is, if you have been using sharps then you clear up what you have used and dispose of them correctly with due consideration for the safety of others.

9 **Spillages** of any kind can be hazardous to your and others' health and wellbeing. The rule is, if you cause the spillage then you clean it up or ensure it is dealt with in the correct way. Your employer's policies and procedures for dealing with spillages must be adhered to at all times.

10 **Waste materials** can be divided into three categories: household, clinical and contaminated/hazardous. However, all categories of waste should be handled with caution as all are capable of increasing the risk of cross infection and causing harm to yourself and others. Your employer's policies and procedures for the disposal of waste must be adhered to at all times.

11 **Linen**, like waste materials, must be handled with care because of the increased potential for cross infection. When handling soiled or contaminated linen appropriate protective clothing should be worn. With regard to the handling of clean linen the *just done, do now* approach should be adopted. Your employer's policies and procedures for the handling of linen must be adhered to at all times.

12 **Food handling** is an activity that all of us do either at a personal level for self-consumption or at a social level for consumption by others. The mishandling of food is a prime source of cross infection and the use of appropriate protective clothing and meticulous hand hygiene is essential using the, *just done, do now* approach.

13 **Environmental contamination**, although not always visible to the human eye, is always present. Therefore, regular and rigorous cleaning of healthcare environments is essential in reducing the risk of cross infection. Although many involved in the provision of healthcare perceive such environmental cleaning as being the role of designated cleaners, such a role is arguably the responsibility of all. The rule is, if you cause the contamination, you clean it up or ensure it is cleaned up in an appropriate manner. It is both unethical and unprofessional to simply leave contamination with the expectation that it is someone else's responsibility to clean it up.

14 **Personal hygiene** of both those involved in the provision of healthcare and

recipients of healthcare is an important measure where the reduction of cross infection is concerned.

Applicants to social work training often state that their main reason for wanting to enter the profession is to help people (Carey 2003). This is an honourable reason, but may, in fact, inhibit effectiveness in certain crucial areas of their role. For example, monitoring or policing poor or harmful practice in themselves or others may be counter-intuitive to the 'benign helper' (*see* Explanation box 9.1).

EXPLANATION BOX 9.1

The concept of the benign helper is drawn from the underlying value base ascribed to helping professionals, including social workers. Although mistakenly thought to have originated in the Hippocratic Oath, the maxim to 'First, do no harm' or '*Primum non nocere*' has been recognised as a guiding principle of doctors, healthcare professionals and social workers alike (Smith 2005). However, I would argue that as members of a caring profession, we are reluctant to recognise that not everything we do will be benign and helpful and understanding that even the most ethical practitioners may cause harm is difficult. We often construct abusive professionals as the 'few rotten apples' in order to maintain a mistaken view that there is possible harm in every intervention we carry out.

   This complexity – that we can both help and harm someone at the same time – induces a very real practice dilemma in the professional (Caplan and Caplan 2001). It may be uncomfortable, but easier to recognise when, for example, giving medical treatment that has unpleasant, harmful or unknown side effects, as long as the potential benefits are also recognised. The process is less clear in terms of psychosocial interventions or in the context of the helping relationship. So, for example, the fact that a reassuring touch of the hand of someone in distress may also be a cause of infection may be a very difficult practice dilemma to resolve.

Understanding or accepting the possibility that social workers may harm a client may at best be restricted to notions of abusive practice as opposed to negligence through non-adherence to standard precautions. Even when considering negligent or poor practice, this may be understood in terms of actions omitted or carried out to a low standard as opposed to impact (Day, Klein and Redmayne 1996). This challenges social workers to think about issues of hand hygiene in a way that may be counter-intuitive to their usual approach to physical proximity and touch. In addition, social workers are used to assessing risk in terms of risk of physical injury to self from or to others as opposed to risk of cross infection.

In terms of infection control, it is well-established that this needs to be a shared responsibility, but it may not always be understood as such. The dominance of health-related jargon, for example HCAI, and substantial guidance being produced by NICE (National Institute for Clinical Excellence) add to the misconception that this is substantially a health professions issue (NICE 2003). There is little similar guidance in social care and that which exists constructs the problem of infection control as being primarily related to social care workers, or those who have direct 'hands on' tasks to perform in residential or nursing home settings or who provide domiciliary personal care (Skills for Care 2005). Education and training on effective infection control is likely to be located at National Vocational Qualification (NVQ) level and is rarely part of a social worker's induction. Likewise, the UK General Social Care Council Codes of Practice for Social Care Workers and Employers does not cover specific aspects of infection control practice, such as standard precautions. However, this could easily be covered under risk assessment and compliance with employers' health and safety policies (General Social Care Council 2002).

REFLECTION EXERCISE 9.3

Think about regular visits you make to individuals in their own homes, in hospital or in care homes.

What are the implications of considering infection control before or after your visit?

Are there some visits where this would 'feel' easier or more appropriate than others?

What are the reasons for this?

Since the implementation in the UK of the National Health Service and Community Care Act (1990) there has been greater emphasis on inter-professional working between health and social services across all adult care sectors, including mental health, learning disability, physical disability and older people (Sharkey 2007). This has led to an increase in the number of social workers and social care workers located alongside health staff in hospitals, general practice surgeries and other clinical settings (Department of Health 2000). However, working effectively inter-professionally presents many challenges for individual staff, managers, policy makers and educators (Charlesworth 2001). Most notable challenges have included reviewing traditional demarcation lines of roles and responsibilities; redefining some previously profession-specific tasks and ensuring maximum effectiveness with neither overlap nor gaps in provision (Glasby and Peck 2004).

In terms of roles and responsibilities, there has been greater clarity of what a social care professional, as opposed to a healthcare professional, is authorised to do by legal definition and by the implementation of regulations specific to social work and social care. From the service user perspective, it is now possible to receive a holistic single assessment of community care and health need as opposed to being subjected to several repetitive assessments by different professionals located in different agencies and buildings. In terms of professional education and training, many universities now provide this at an undergraduate pre-registration level on an inter-professional basis.

However, the need for a joined-up approach to infection control has not yet gained significant attention in the current debates and this is a worrying omission. For example, the National Service Framework (NSF) for Older People (Department of Health 2001) states in its introduction that it

> . . . sets new national standards and service models of care across health and social services for all older people, whether they live at home, in residential care or are being looked after in hospital.

It aims to tackle age discrimination, health promotion in later life, support a coordinated approach to person-centred care – whether in hospital or community settings – and also to strokes, falls and mental health. It does not mention the need for a coordinated approach to infection control (*see* Explanation box 9.2).

EXPLANATION BOX 9.2

In the UK, there have been many criticisms of health and social care provision, which historically was provided by separate organisations, funded by separate budgets and characterised by a divided approach. Failures in the system were highlighted by high-profile cases involving mentally ill patients in the community who either put themselves at unacceptable risk (McFadyen and Farrington 1996) or who became a danger to the public (Ritchie, Dick and Lingham 1994). Since then, government policy has supported the integration of health and social care services and its practice has developed into a more integrated or joined-up approach. However, current agendas have focused on areas such as care of the mentally ill, discharge planning for older people, adult protection, partnership with service users and carers and specialisations such as palliative care and dementia. The need to apply this joined-up or partnership approach to infection control has not yet been recognised as a significant area for exploration.

In addition, the issue of hand hygiene (which is raised in one of the first inter-professional pre-registration modules at Canterbury Christ Church University) is the topic most often complained about as being of no relevance to first year social work students and is often characterised as a nursing issue. These assumptions are based on false notions that infections are spread in hospital settings only, that nurses are the only profession who work in hospital settings, and that social workers do not undertake any 'hands on' tasks and therefore are immune from, or not part of, the infection-control chain (*see* Explanation box 9.3).

EXPLANATION BOX 9.3

In the UK, there are areas of personal caring that social workers may not undertake because the law does not permit it, such as giving injections or changing certain dressings. However, there are also areas of work which, because they are traditionally carried out by social care or domiciliary workers, have not formed part of a social worker role. These areas are not defined by statute or law, but are often crudely described as 'hands on' care and that is how I use the term here.

These assumptions must be challenged in both the learning environment and practice. For example, whilst social workers may not see their role as being primarily to offer personal care, there are many situations where their hands may come into contact with a service user.

REFLECTION EXERCISE 9.4

Personal care can be identified as

> . . . care that directly involves touching a person's body, and is distinct from treatment/therapy – a procedure that is deliberately intended to cure or

ameliorate a pathological condition – and from indirect care, such as home help or the provision of meals on wheels (Royal Commission on Long-term Care 1999, p. 67).

Consider what is meant by personal care by the definition above.

Social workers do not carry out physical interventions or treatment, but think about in what way might you touch a client?
Do you shake hands when you introduce yourself?
Do you offer a helping hand on someone's arm if they have a mobility issue?
Do you offer a hand in reassurance if someone is upset?
Do you help someone on or off with their outdoor clothes when taking them somewhere?
Are there other examples?

Should you consider infection control in any of these examples?
How would you manage that?
What would you say to your client about it?

Working inter-professionally requires practitioners to be able to maintain strong individual professional identities and clear demarcation lines about certain roles and tasks whilst understanding the complexity of what might be shared or interchangeable tasks (Brown, Crawford and Darongkamas 2000). For example, whilst a mental health social worker may monitor the compliance of a patient with their monthly depot injection, they are never in a position to administer that injection (Dougherty and Lister 2004). Therefore, their task is perceived as being at a physical distance to the client even though there may be a physical treatment issue involved. In contrast, practitioners need to adopt a shared approach with certain tasks. Some such roles and tasks include assessment of need, care planning, coordination of care and reviewing of care. In other circumstances, tasks can be allocated to a single professional who represents the inter-professional team, such as liaising with carers, discharge planning or referring to their agencies. These different approaches make certain areas of responsibility explicit and clearly attributable, but tasks such as infection control may not have sufficient clarity. In addition, practitioners have been encouraged to minimise the overlap or duplication of tasks and it has therefore become counter-intuitive to do otherwise. Working inter-professionally and safely from an infection-control perspective requires not only an understanding of the distinct and shared roles, but also perhaps a duplication and repetition of tasks. Reflecting on both the implications and challenges of this counter-intuitive approach can be a useful way of addressing dangerous practices.

The responsibility for infection control in inter-professional teams is not always clearly understood or articulated, particularly when the team is involved in the psychosocial care of clients or patients (Gammon, Morgan-Samuel and Gould 2008). As with difficult patients or clients, there is a danger that it is seen as an issue no one wants and is therefore passed around the team to the person who is least able to resist the pressure to take responsibility. However, there are clearly dangers in this approach as there are occasions when patients fall through the net.

REFLECTION EXERCISE 9.5

Consider the list below and reflect on who you believe is responsible for infection control. Do any of the professions/roles below not have responsibility? Do some of these professions/roles have more responsibility than others? If so why?

Service managers	Doctors
Hospital nurses	Community nurses
Care workers	Social workers
Ancillary staff: porters, cleaners	Administrators/reception staff
Volunteers	Patients/clients
Visitors or friends of patients/clients	Ambulance crews
Dentists	Dental nurses

Now identify whether infection control should be profession- or role-specific, a shared role or an interchangeable role.

Of the above professions/roles, who do you believe is most responsible for cross infection? Now think about your answer and ask yourself the question, 'Is my answer rational or rationalised?'

Vulnerable people have always been accommodated in a variety of in-patient and community settings. This is not a new phenomenon. However, the landscape of coordinated community care has changed and consequently there is a need to widen responsibility for infection control to a broader range of contexts (Skills for Care 2005). For example, there has been an increase in the number of minor operations carried out in general practice surgeries (Brown *et al.* 1997). In addition, patients or clients are being discharged into the community, to their own homes or to supported living, residential or nursing home care, as soon as they are deemed medically fit for discharge (Baumann *et al.* 2007). This is reflected in the changing context of social work practice and the degree to which social workers in adult care are now firmly established as care managers (Brown, Crawford and Darongkamas 2000). Alongside this, previously hidden groups of patients or clients have emerged. For example, victims of adult abuse, carers, people living with HIV and AIDS – social workers need to take a holistic approach to their needs too.

Planning smooth care pathways and ensuring seamless services between health and social care are the new priorities, but this has not always been the core social work role and is not necessarily welcomed by some current practitioners. Care managers have reported feeling that their profession has become bureaucratised and that this has led to a restriction on their ability to make meaningful and empowering relationships with their clients (Carey 2003; Tanner 1998). For example, having additional procedures to follow to implement infection control may not be welcome in the current climate and may be wrongly perceived as the antithesis of core social work practice. It may also be perceived as a direct result of the implementation of the NHS and Community Care Act (1990) and as such the ambivalence surrounding those imposed changes may impact on a practitioner's willingness to proactively engage with the issue. Furthermore, infection control procedures may not sit comfortably alongside other care management or social work tasks and may be rejected, or their importance diminished, if they are perceived as increasing this bureaucratisation.

REFLECTION EXERCISE 9.6

Think about the different roles/tasks you perform during your working day as a health or social care professional.

Make a list of the roles or tasks you like doing the most.
  Which are the ones you least like?
  Where would you place infection control in relation to the roles or tasks you like doing most and those you like doing least?

Do you consider infection control as a part of following essential procedures (just something else you have to do) or part of establishing and maintaining safe and meaningful relationships with your patients or clients?

It is often assumed that safe, meaningful relationships between social workers and their clients are at the heart of much social work practice where the possibility of therapeutic change exists (Beresford, Croft and Adshead 2007; Parry-Jones *et al.*1998). Such areas of work include work with children, therapeutic work with survivors of abuse or trauma, or counselling people through loss or bereavement.

However, safe and meaningful relationships are considered less often where the possibility of therapeutic change appears less likely. This includes work with older people, people with dementia, learning disabilities or long-term conditions or illnesses. There is a growing body of concern that social workers are failing to see the opportunities to apply their skills in a person-centred way in these areas. For example, living with dementia involves multiple losses for the individual and their family and friends. The condition usually progresses slowly over a considerable period of time and could provide many opportunities for therapeutic work on loss. Unfortunately, this psychotherapeutic intervention is rarely offered or considered when care management priorities and work load pressures restrict the time social workers have available.

Social work tasks are driven by planning care within restrictive budgets and the importance of the interaction or relationship between social worker and client has become secondary. The erosion of this part of a social work role does not help in the implementation of infection control if the main aim is perceived as undertaking bureaucratic tasks as speedily and efficiently as possible.

REFLECTION EXERCISE 9.7

Consider the following statement:

> 'Social workers and care managers do not have time to implement relevant standard precautions of infection control.'

As a social work professional, how do you feel about this?
As a healthcare professional, how do you feel about this?
What are the reasons for feeling this way?
What are the implications of this?
What can you, as an individual, do about this?

Working with human beings in severe distress can be a source of disabling anxiety for health and social care professionals (Menzies-Lyth 1988). However, a crucial part of the role of practitioners is to contain anxiety for their clients, as well as managing their own. Social workers are being increasingly encouraged to not only use reflection as a way of developing critical practice, but also as a means to gain insight into these anxiety-laden interpersonal processes they engage in with their clients (Ruch 2007). Therefore, holistic reflection can be usefully employed to understand the anxieties inherent in social work practice relating to infection control. The availability of safe arenas for discussion and reflection are essential for the containment of anxiety.

REFLECTION EXERCISE 9.8

Think about the anxieties you may have about infection control; for example:
● remembering the standard precautions;
● feeling worried about personal contact with clients;
● feeling worried about how to speak with a client about infection control;
● any others?

Think about arenas where you might discuss anxieties about infection control. Which arenas would feel the safest:
    Individual supervision?
    Team meetings?
    Multi-professional meetings?
    Informal contact with colleagues?
Which arenas would help you to manage your own anxiety?

CONCLUSION

It is a core social work task to adhere to appropriate standard precautions (*see* List 9.1) in the area of infection control. It is important for social workers to be informed about these standard precautions and how to apply them effectively. However, it is also important for social workers to reflect upon barriers to their effective implementation. It is critical that social workers recognise the issue as one of effective partnership in working with health colleagues; as one which draws on their ability to effectively assess risk; as an issue related to ethical behaviour and personal/professional boundaries and one where social workers' knowledge and skills around inequality and empowerment may be crucial.

REFERENCES

Baumann M, Evans S, Perkins M, *et al.* Organisation and features of hospital, intermediate care and social services in English sites with low rates of delayed discharge. *Health Soc Care Comm.* 2007; **15**(4): 295–305.

Beresford P, Croft S, Adshead L. 'We don't see her as a social worker': a service user case study of the importance of the social worker's relationship and humanity. *Brit J Soc Work.* 2008 **38**: 1388–407.

Brown B, Crawford P, Darongkamas J. Blurred roles and permeable boundaries: the experience of multidisciplinary working in community mental health. *Health Soc Care Comm.* 2000; **8**(6): 425–35.

Brown JS, Smith RR. Cantor T, *et al.* General practitioners as providers of minor surgery: a success story? *Brit J Gen Pract.* 1997; **47**(417): 205–10.

Caplan C, Caplan RB. *Helping the Helpers Not to Harm: iatrogenic damage and community mental health.* New York: Brunner Routledge; 2001.

Carey M. Anatomy of a care manager. *Work Employ Soc.* 2003; **17**(1): 121–35.

Charlesworth J. Negotiating and managing partnerships in primary care. *Health Soc Care Comm.* 2001; **9**(5): 279–85.

Day P, Klein R, Redmayne S. *Why Regulate?: regulating residential care for elderly people.* Bristol: The Policy Press; 1996.

D'Cruz H, Gillingham P, Melendez S. Reflexivity: its meanings and relevance for social work: a critical review of the literature. *Br J Soc Work.* 2007; **37**: 73–90.

Department of Health. *NHS and Community Care Act.* London: Department of Health; 1990.

Department of Health. *The NHS Plan.* London: Department of Health; 2000.

Department of Health. *National Service Framework for Older People.* London: Department of Health; 2001.

Dougherty L, Lister S, editors. *The Royal Marsden Hospital Manual of Clinical Nursing Procedures.* 6th ed. Oxford: Blackwell Publishing; 2004.

Gammon J, Morgan-Samuel H, Gould D. A review of the evidence for suboptimal compliance of healthcare practitioners to standard/universal infection control precautions. *J Clin Nurs.* 2008; **17**(2): 157–67.

General Social Care Council. *Codes of Practice for Social Care Workers and Employers.* London: General Social Care Council; 2002.

Glasby J, Peck E, editors. *Care Trusts: partnership working in action.* Oxford: Radcliffe Publishing; 2004.

McFadyen J, Farrington A. Mental healthcare in the community. *Pract Nurs.* 1996; **7**(15): 32–4.

Menzies-Lyth I. *Containing Anxiety in Institutions: selected essays.* Vol. 1. London: Free Association Books; 1988.

National Institute for Clinical Excellence. *Infection Control: prevention of healthcare-associated infection in primary and community care.* London: National Institute for Clinical Excellence; 2003.

Parry-Jones B, Grant G, McGrath M, *et al.* Stress and job satisfaction among social workers, community nurses and community psychiatric nurses: implications for the care management model. *Health Soc Care Comm.* 1998; **6**(4): 271–85.

Ritchie JH, Dick D, Lingham R. *The Report of the Inquiry into the Care and Treatment of Christopher Clunis.* London: HMSO; 1994.

Royal Commission on Long-term Care. *With Respect to Old Age: long-term care – rights and responsibilities.* London: HMSO; 1999.

Ruch G. Reflective practice in contemporary child-care social work: the role of containment. *Br J Soc Work.* 2007; **37**: 659–80.

Saltiel D. Teaching reflective research and practice on a post qualifying child care programme. *Soc Work Educ.* 2003; **22**(1): 105–11.

Schön D. *The Reflective Practitioner.* 2nd ed. Aldershot: Arena; 1991.

Sharkey P. *The Essentials of Community Care.* 2nd ed. Basingstoke: Palgrave Macmillan; 2007.

Skills for Care. *Knowledge Set for Infection Prevention and Control.* Leeds: Skills for Care; 2005.

Smith CM. Origin and uses of *Primum non nocere*: above all do no harm. *J Clin Pharmacol.* 2005; **45**: 371–7.

Tanner D. Empowerment and care management: swimming against the tide. *Health Soc Care Comm.* 1998; **6**(6): 447–57.

Washer P, Joffe H. The 'hospital superbug': social representations of MRSA. *Soc Sci Med.* 2006; **63**(8): 2141–52.

CHAPTER 10

Clinical supervision as a facilitator of safe practice

CLINICAL SUPERVISION

➤ What is it?
➤ What does the term mean?
➤ What is it supposed to do?
➤ How can it be applied to infection control as a strategy for enhancing adherence to standard precautions?

Within this chapter it is my intention to reflect upon all of these questions with the aim of demonstrating that, if used appropriately, clinical supervision can be a powerful force in reducing non-adherence to standard precautions. I will do this from two broad perspectives: terminology and models. Terminology will involve reflecting upon the terms 'clinical supervision', 'person-centred development' (Elliott cited in Jasper 2006), 'supervisor', 'supervisee', 'facilitator' and 'recipient'. A number of models will be reflected upon regarding their suitability as facilitators of personal and professional development. Both standpoints will be linked to their potential for reducing non-adherence to standard precautions among health and social care professionals.

TERMINOLOGY

What does the term 'clinical supervision' mean to you?

How do you feel it could be used to enhance adherence to standard precautions?

In thinking about the questions in Reflection exercise 10.1, you may have reached two conclusions. Firstly, that the term 'clinical supervision' is inappropriate; and when measured against the concept of person-centred development (Elliott cited in Jasper 2006) it will be unlikely to facilitate improved adherence to standard precautions. Bond and Holland (1998) provide a definition of clinical supervision as 'regular, protected time for facilitated, in-depth reflection on clinical practice' (p. 12). If we draw out the key words of this definition and

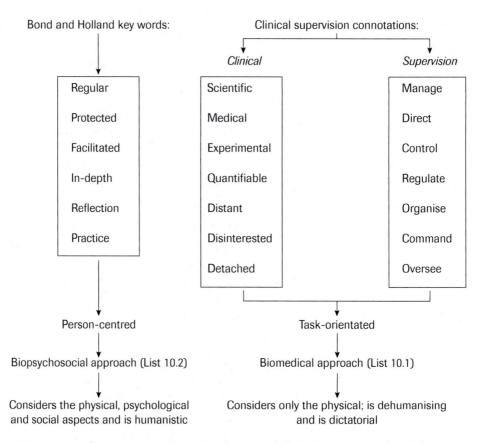

FIGURE 10.1 A comparison between the term 'clinical supervision' and Bond and Holland's (1999) definition of the term.

compare them with the words 'clinical' and 'supervision' (*see* Figure 10.1) it becomes very evident that the two are completely incompatible.

Therefore, because clinical supervision is an anomaly in that it indicates one thing but means another, if it is to be used as a method for enhancing adherence to standard precautions we must firstly determine an alternative term that reflects the concept where one individual (the supervisor) facilitates the personal and professional development of one or more individuals (the supervisee/s) through a reflective exchange (Howatson-Jones 2003). Secondly, we must expand upon the definition identified by Bond and Holland (1998) because arguably the complexity of the clinical supervision process is such that it cannot be defined in a single sentence. Therefore, in determining an alternative for 'clinical supervision' that will enhance the potential for reducing non-adherence to standard precautions, let us consider the term within the context of the biomedical (*see* List 10.1) and biopsychosocial (*see* List 10.2) approaches.

LIST 10.1 A BIOMEDICAL APPROACH TO CLINICAL SUPERVISION

Here are examples of where a biomedical approach to clinical supervision is used:

- An individual's supervisor is chosen for them.
- Clinical supervision is forced upon individuals.
- Clinical supervision is about managing and controlling individuals.
- A supervisor's role is to tell individuals what they must do.
- Clinical supervision is a way of spying on individuals.
- Clinical supervision is a means of organisations achieving their corporate objectives.
- Ethical and human rights issues are irrelevant (*see* List 10.3).
- A supervisor's role is to promote dissonance-based thinking (*see* Explanation box 10.1), cognitively economic perspectives (*see* Explanation box 10.2) and unrealistically optimistic beliefs (*see* Explanation box 10.3).
- Conflict should be encouraged between the supervisor and supervisee(s) or between supervisees.
- Supervisors can use conflict between supervisees as a means of control; i.e. divide and conquer.
- Stress and anxiety are a normal part of receiving clinical supervision.
- Clinical supervision should be based upon an external locus of control (*see* Explanation box 10.4).
- Clinical supervision has nothing to do with personal and professional

development unless it is consistent with an employer's needs.
- Clinical supervision exists to allow a supervisor to impose their views upon the supervisee(s).
- Clinical supervision should be used to depersonalise, stereotype and deny freedom of choice.

LIST 10.2 A BIOPSYCHOSOCIAL APPROACH TO CLINICAL SUPERVISION

Here are examples of where a biopsychosocial approach to clinical supervision is used:
- Clinical supervision is about recognising that within the process there will always be physical, psychological and social issues.
- Individuals have the right to choose their supervisor.
- Within the clinical supervision process all are equal, including the supervisor.
- The role of supervisor is that of a facilitator and to manage or control.
- The role of the supervisor is to challenge and promote the supervisee(s) critical reflection skills.
- The supervisor's role is to facilitate the individual in becoming aware of and confronting their dissonance-based thinking (see Explanation box 10.1), cognitively economic perspectives (see Explanation box 10.2) and unrealistically optimistic beliefs (see Explanation box 10.3).
- The clinical supervision process should promote the idea of freedom of choice, freedom of thought and freedom of expression within a secure and confidential atmosphere.
- Clinical supervision has nothing to do with corporate objectives, but has everything to do with an individual's personal and professional development. However, the astute supervisor will recognise that facilitating an individual's personal and professional development will indirectly support the achievement of corporate objectives.
- Successful clinical supervision has everything to do with ensuring the needs of the supervisee(s) are met and human rights are maintained.
- Ensuring an ethical approach is central to the success of clinical supervision.
- Challenging debate and discussion are fundamental to successful clinical supervision.
- Clinical supervision is intended to facilitate the supervisee(s) in reducing

any stress or anxiety they are experiencing.
- The clinical supervision process should be reflective of an internal locus of control (*see* Explanation box 10.4).
- Clinical supervision is not about one individual imposing their views. Rather, it is about a free flow of ideas and feelings between those present.
- Clinical supervision is about respecting the views, feelings and ideas of others – even if they differ from yours.

From reading the content of these two lists and comparing them with Figure 10.1, it is clear that if clinical supervision is to enhance adherence to standard precautions it must be undertaken in a person-centred way and follow a biopsychosocial approach. However, if a biomedical approach is followed, not only will clinical supervision be task-orientated and dictatorial but will also have the propensity to breach the human rights of those involved (*see* List 10.3).

EXPLANATION BOX 10.1 COGNITIVE DISSONANCE (FESTINGER 1962)

The concept of cognitive dissonance was originally identified by Festinger (1962), where he proposed that, at a psychological level, the individual will strive to make consistent two or more things that would not naturally be so. In simple terms, dissonance effects are when an individual generates excuses to justify their previous behaviour or behaviour they wish or intend to carry out. Hand hygiene is a good example, where the individual understands its importance in reducing cross infection, yet fails to adequately follow the hand hygiene process. Thus the individual experiences conflict between knowing what they should do and what they actually do or want to do.

Such conflict would manifest as stress in the individual and in an attempt to reduce such stress the individual will generate an excuse or reason for failing to follow the hand hygiene process. Such an excuse may be blamed on time, work load or an irrational belief that meeting other's needs must take priority.

EXPLANATION BOX 10.2 COGNITIVE ECONOMY
(ROTH AND FRISBY 1992)

Cognitive economy is where an individual has become context-specific or tunnel-visioned in their perception of what is occurring around them and will fail to take into account the wider implications of their behaviour. For example, instead of being patient-centred, the individual will become task-orientated towards achieving a set of goals that will meet their own needs at the expense of everything else and the needs of others.

Example: In the case of standard precautions, the individual will be context-specific towards achieving their allocated work load and as a result of this may:

- fail to change their gloves between interventions;
- fail to undertake or to fully follow the hand hygiene process;
- fail to ensure that they have removed all the equipment they used following completion of a procedure.

EXPLANATION BOX 10.3 UNREALISTIC OPTIMISM (OGDEN 2007)

Unrealistic optimism is where a health or social care professional becomes unrealistically optimistic regarding the risky situation they place themselves and others in as a result of behaviour that constitutes unsafe infection control practice in the form of failing to undertake standard precautions or through failing to follow the hand hygiene process.

Unrealistic optimism can be facilitated through lack of personal experience. For example, a health or social care professional who has no prior experience of a patient's or client's health being directly influenced by their failure to adopt appropriate standard precautions will likely believe two things (Elliott 2003):

1 There is no risk, or the risk of cross infecting others is so insignificant that it simply does not matter.

2 Even if there is a risk it will not happen to them. That is, even if the individual involved in healthcare does cross infect others they will rationalise that is was not their fault (*see* Explanation box 10.1) or they will not be found out and held responsible and therefore, who cares?

EXPLANATION BOX 10.4 HEALTH LOCUS OF CONTROL (WALLSTON AND WALLSTON 1982; ADAMS AND BROMLEY 1998)

Locus of control consists of two dimensions:

1 Internal: This is the partnership between the patient or client and the health-care worker, whether it be professional, administrative, managerial or ancillary. Such partnerships reflect the provision of information, non-judgemental attitudes and the right to ask questions without fear of ridicule and retribution. Such an approach is reflective of a biopsychosocial perspective.

Example: With regard to standard precautions, patients and clients have the right to have their questions answered in order for them to make informed choices as to whether they wish to comply with the advice given by healthcare workers.

2   External: This is where the patient or client is expected to be unquestioning, compliant and submissive to the demands of healthcare workers. Such an approach is reflective of a biomedical perspective.

Example: With regard to standard precautions, patients and clients are denied the opportunity to ensure that these are appropriately applied within the context of their healthcare experience.

LIST 10.3 CLINICAL SUPERVISION AND HUMAN RIGHTS INFRINGEMENTS

The following are examples of how clinical supervision could infringe an individual's human rights (Elliott cited in Jasper 2006; Wilkinson and Caulfield 2001). However, the items noted below should not be seen as being mutually exclusive, but as offering a perspective.

Article 1 – Obligations to secure rights and freedoms: An individual has the right to receive clinical supervision if they wish. An individual cannot be forced to take clinical supervision just because a manager or employer decides to implement it. If an individual is forced to take clinical supervision against their wishes then they could argue that their human rights have been infringed.

Article 3 – Prohibition of torture: If a manager or employer forces or coerces an individual to take clinical supervision against their will and as such they experience stress and anxiety then that individual might argue that their human rights have been infringed as a result of a given manager or employer causing them to suffer a torturous psychological or social experience. For example:

- Psychological torture could result from the emotional distress the individual might experience as a result of being forced to do something against their will.
- Social torture could result from being forced to take clinical supervision with a supervisor who they did not choose, with whom they do not feel comfortable with and with whom they are concerned about communicating openly with for fear of the supervisor divulging what the supervisee says.

Article 8 – The right to respect for private and family life: Within a clinical supervision session, an individual has the right to have what they say respected and not to feel forced or pressured into discussing issues that they feel will infringe upon their privacy. If an individual feels their privacy has not been respected or maintained then they might argue that their human rights have been infringed.

Article 9 – Freedom of thought, conscience and religion: Within a clinical supervision session, every individual present has the right to convey their thoughts, feelings and beliefs without fear of ridicule or retribution regarding topics being reflected upon. If an individual within a clinical supervision session is denied this right then they might argue that their human rights have been infringed.

Article 10 – Freedom of expression: Within clinical supervision sessions, individuals have the right to express their opinions and to receive appropriate information in a non-judgemental or prejudicial manner. If an individual is not afforded this freedom then they might argue that their human rights have been infringed.

Article 11 – Freedom of assembly and association: If an individual chooses to meet on a regular basis with another individual or individuals and apply the philosophies that underpin clinical supervision as a means of facilitating personal and professional development, and they are prevented from doing this by a manager or employer, provided that such a meeting does not infringe upon patient or client care or the conditions set out within their contract of employment then that individual or individuals might argue that their human rights have been infringed. However, an astute manager or employer would recognise the value of such meetings and as such actively facilitate their occurrence.

Unfortunately it is a sad reflection that many employers and professions approach clinical supervision from a biomedical perspective and perceive it as a means of monitoring and controlling individuals with regard to their professional activities. It is for this reason that clinical supervision so often fails and is rejected by individuals. Clinical supervision must therefore be re-titled.

The re-titling of any term that has become institutionalised, as is the case with 'clinical supervision', will be problematic. This is because such an institutionalised term will have become jargonised within common language. Therefore, getting health and social care professionals to adopt a different term would involve a change in the way they think, and as we have identified within previous chapters, changing the way individuals think is, at best, difficult and especially so if the term we wish to change has become widespread and universal. Because of this, the new term needs to meet five criteria:

1 The need to be orientated towards the individual.

2 The need to provide a clear focus.
3 The need to reflect achievement and progress.
4 The need to be consistent with the philosophies set down within codes of conduct and positive working practices.
5 The need to carry universal meaning.

Therefore the term 'person-centred development' (Elliott cited in Jasper 2006) would be more appropriate because the word *person* is consistent with points 1, 2, 3 and 5 (above); the word *centred* is consistent with points 1, 2, 3 and 5 and the word *development* is consistent with points 2, 3, 4 and 5.

REFLECTION EXERCISE 10.2

Take some time to think about the two terms 'clinical supervision' and 'person-centred development'.

Which do you think is more appropriate when measured against the breakdown of Bond and Holland's definition (*see* Figure 10.1)?

In replacing the term 'clinical supervision' with 'person-centred development', I would argue the latter is consistent with the definition set out by Bond and Holland (1998) (*see* Figure 10.1); is consistent with an internal locus of control (*see* Explanation box 10.4); is reflective of a biopsychosocial approach (*see* List 10.2) and as such will provide a catalyst for reducing non-adherence to standard precautions.

The importance of having an appropriate catalyst is vital because without it an individual's interpretation of the process will be affected. For example, the first step in using person-centred development as a means of reducing non-adherence to standard precautions depends upon what people perceive person-centred development to be. Using the term 'clinical supervision' will create negative connotations (*see* Figure 10.1). For example, it can give the impression that 'Management are at it again; they just want to keep an eye on what we are doing'. Therefore individuals will be likely to interpret the process as being consistent with a biomedical approach (*see* List 10.1) and an external locus of control (*see* Explanation box 10.4). Such an interpretation will inhibit an individual's motivation towards undertaking clinical supervision. In contrast, if the term 'person-centred development' is used, it will serve to facilitate positive connotations of the process (*see* List 10.2). For example, it gives the impression that 'This is for me and about me', which should help to motivate individuals towards finding out more. In attempting to find out

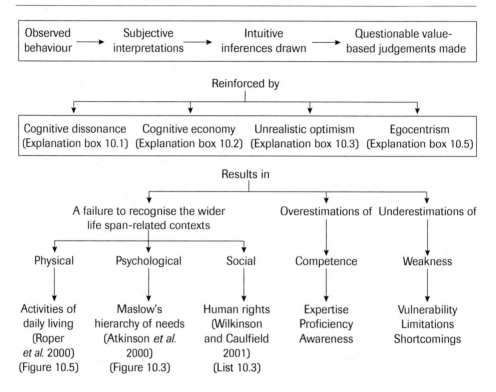

FIGURE 10.2 Observational judgement.

more, the primary motivator will be 'What's in it for me'? The outcome of this should be to instil within the individual the feeling that in undertaking person-centred development:

➤ They will be supported.
➤ They will be valued.
➤ The process will help them to reduce their stress.
➤ The process will enhance their self-confidence.
➤ The process will enhance their self-esteem.
➤ The process will enhance their self-awareness with regard to:
   — the quality of their infection control practice;
   — areas of their practice that require improvement;
   — areas of their practice that are positive;
   — the impact psychosocial factors can have upon their adherence to standard precautions.
➤ The process will facilitate their ability to reflect both in and upon practice.
➤ The process will enhance their ability to develop both personally and professionally.

➤ The process will facilitate them in recognising their achievements and in actively promoting those achievements to others.
➤ The process will in part be owned by them.

However, having identified the value of a title change intended to facilitate personal and professional development, the question must be posed, 'Is it enough to simply state a change of title is needed?' The simple answer to this is 'No'.

REFLECTION EXERCISE 10.3

Why is it not enough to say something must change?
    What would have to be done or demonstrated to your satisfaction that the term 'clinical supervision' should be changed to 'person-centred development'?

Bearing in mind that the term 'clinical supervision' has become a jargonised aspect of common language within health and social care, it is necessary to provide some validity for making such a change. In attempting to offer a valid reason for this change, I refer you back to the differences between the biomedical and biopsychosocial approaches (*see* Lists 10.1 and 10.2). Clearly, clinical supervision is consistent with the biomedical approach and is about exerting power, coercion and control. However, the biopsychosocial approach places the person (supervisee) at the centre of the process and gives control of that process to them. Therefore, a good facilitator of person-centred development will adopt a biopsychosocial approach. A bad facilitator will adopt a biomedical approach.

MODELS

If person-centred development is to reduce non-adherence to standard precautions, there must also be a review of the models that are advocated as being suitable to follow. Currently, there are a number of models in existence that are supposed to promote the process of person-centred development. However, as these models are referred to within the context of clinical supervision they will have the potential to fail in facilitating improved adherence to standard precautions. For example, a model linked with the term 'clinical supervision' and a model linked with the term 'person-centred development' will cause an individual to think about them differently. Furthermore, the title given to a model will also impact upon what an individual believes a given model is about. Changing the name does not change the nature of the model. For example, the integrated and orientation-specific models (Leddick 1994) and the cognitive therapy supervision model (Sloan and Watson 2002) will cause an individual to make inferred judgements about those models. However, the inferred judgements we make are not necessarily a true reflection of a model's intention. Therefore titling is important.

Integrated model

In considering the integrated model, the role of the facilitator (supervisor) is to lecture and instruct the participant (supervisee). Yet to lecture and instruct is simply not consistent with the philosophy of person-centred development or a biopsychosocial approach (*see* List 10.2). They are more consistent with managing, controlling, dictating and a biomedical approach (*see* List 10.1).

Orientation-specific model

The orientation-specific model centres around the facilitator (supervisor) and recipient (supervisee) observing each other's competence and weaknesses and then using what they have inferred from their observations to attribute influence and authority over the other person. This stance is not consistent with the philosophy of person-centred development or a biopsychosocial approach. However, it is again consistent with the ideas of controlling and dictating and a biomedical approach.

Furthermore, the principle of observation, which appears to be a criterion that underpins this model, makes it very questionable when examined within the context of the reliability of human observation. As we have already identified in Chapter 7, what we interpret from our observations can be easily fooled. Any model that promotes the idea of observation determining absolutes upon which reliable judgements can be made should be discarded without delay. As such, any model that relies upon observation as a catalyst for reducing non-adherence to standard precautions will be destined to fail because each individual has their own beliefs about what constitutes appropriate adherence to standard precautions. Therefore, in observing a colleague's adoption of standard precautions, their judgement will be based upon subjective interpretation and intuitive inferences (*see* Figure 10.2).

Cognitive therapy model

Although the cognitive therapy model acknowledges that the process should be focused, educational and collaborative, it also indicates that the process should be structured and have a predetermined agenda.

Consider the advantages and disadvantages of making person-centred development sessions structured with a predetermined agenda.

Do you think being structured with a predetermined agenda could be reflective of a biomedical approach (*see* List 10.1) and an external locus of control (*see* Explanation box 10.4)?

Who do you think would benefit more from your person-centred development session: you or the supervisor?

In considering structure and predetermined agendas, we need to pose the question, 'Who are these more likely to serve best?' One of the philosophies that underpins person-centred development is the idea that within sessions all those involved hold equal status, irrespective of their profession, role or appointment, including the session facilitator (supervisor). In addition, it will, to a greater extent, be difficult to predict the content and nature of any discussion that may occur during a session. Discussion within one session may or may not be a reflection of discussions that took place within previous sessions. However, attempting to take a structured approach and to set predetermined agendas for sessions may well restrict the quality and diversity of interaction and discussion. Therefore, structuring and setting of predetermined agendas are consistent with forcing or directing what will be discussed, and could lead to one individual being able to impose their views. This is reflective of managing and controlling (*see* List 10.1) and can lead to human rights infringements (*see* List 10.3).

The cognitive therapy model also draws a link between treatment and supervision. I would argue that the drawing of such links is dangerous and assumes that those undertaking person-centred development not only need to be managed and controlled, but also require some form of treatment or therapy, which are all consistent with a biomedical approach (*see* List 10.1). However, this is not consistent with the philosophy of person-centred development or a biopsychosocial approach (*see* List 10.2) or the maintenance of an individual's human rights (*see* List 10.3). Just because an individual chooses to undertake person-centred development does not mean they are in need of therapy or treatment.

The integrated model, the orientation-specific model and the cognitive therapy model should never be applied within a person-centred development setting and would undoubtedly have a destructive effect. However, it is perhaps because such models have been applied in the past that many within health and social care have misinterpreted what person-centred

EXPLANATION BOX 10.5 DEFINING EGOCENTRIC/EGOCENTRISM

Within the context of Freud's model of the psyche (Freud 1933 in Slack 1981) egocentrism would be reflective of functioning at an Id level.

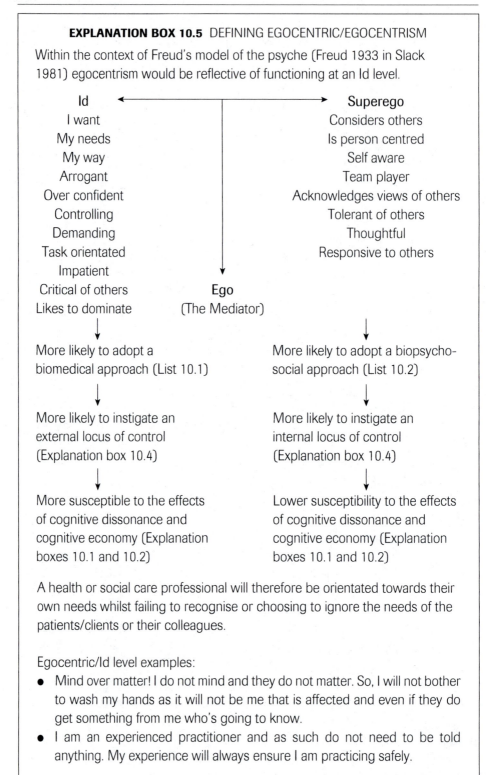

Id		Superego
I want		Considers others
My needs		Is person centred
My way		Self aware
Arrogant		Team player
Over confident		Acknowledges views of others
Controlling		Tolerant of others
Demanding		Thoughtful
Task orientated		Responsive to others
Impatient		
Critical of others	Ego	
Likes to dominate	(The Mediator)	

More likely to adopt a biomedical approach (List 10.1)

More likely to adopt a biopsycho-social approach (List 10.2)

More likely to instigate an external locus of control (Explanation box 10.4)

More likely to instigate an internal locus of control (Explanation box 10.4)

More susceptible to the effects of cognitive dissonance and cognitive economy (Explanation boxes 10.1 and 10.2)

Lower susceptibility to the effects of cognitive dissonance and cognitive economy (Explanation boxes 10.1 and 10.2)

A health or social care professional will therefore be orientated towards their own needs whilst failing to recognise or choosing to ignore the needs of the patients/clients or their colleagues.

Egocentric/Id level examples:
- Mind over matter! I do not mind and they do not matter. So, I will not bother to wash my hands as it will not be me that is affected and even if they do get something from me who's going to know.
- I am an experienced practitioner and as such do not need to be told anything. My experience will always ensure I am practicing safely.

development (clinical supervision) is really about, and as a consequence, have rejected the idea of undertaking it. Such models may also have impacted upon individuals' motivation to undertake person-centred development because some employers and professions have used them inappropriately as controlling, monitoring or manipulation mechanisms. Within the context of infection control, such models will never be successful in reducing non-adherence to standard precautions. In fact, they will be more likely to increase non-adherence through enhancing the effects of cognitive dissonance (*see* Explanation box 10.1), cognitive economy (*see* Explanation box 10.2) and unrealistic optimism (*see* Explanation box 10.3).

For example, observation-based models, by virtue of their propensity to produce unreliable interpretations of others' competence levels and weaknesses, will lead to rationalised (*see* Explanation box 10.1), as opposed to rational, judgements regarding a given individual's competence in adhering to standard precautions. Such rationalised judgements will be the result of a cognitively economic perspective (*see* Explanation box 10.2). That is, the observer will judge competence according to their beliefs and expectations regarding what constitutes appropriate adherence to standard precautions. Therefore an individual's interpretations will have resulted from intuitive inferences whilst failing to consider the wider context (*see* Figure 10.2). Furthermore, cognitive dissonance (*see* Explanation box 10.1) and tunnel-vision (*see* Explanation box 10.2) effects will make the individual unrealistically optimistic (*see* Explanation box 10.3) regarding their judgements about others' competence levels and weaknesses.

REFLECTION EXERCISE 10.5

Consider why you might be overly optimistic about a colleague's adherence to standard precautions.

For example, if the colleague is your friend and you knew that by telling them their adherence to standard precautions was dangerous and unacceptable you would damage or end your friendship, would you still tell them? Who would you put first, the patients/clients or your friend? Be honest!

In being unrealistically optimistic you would be highly likely to cause an individual to make serious over- or under-estimations of others (Engle cited in Skevington 1996). Your estimations would be heavily influenced by your relationship with the other person, whether or not you liked them, your interpretation of their professional standing, their gender, whether you found them attractive or not and what others have told you about them. The adoption of biomedically orientated approaches and observation models by facilitators (supervisors) as a framework for improving adherence to standard precautions within a person-centred development context will be destined to dangerous failure.

At this point I would like to reflect on the terminology that is currently in use. As I have already argued, the term 'clinical supervision' should be changed to 'person-centred development'. I would also offer the same argument for the words 'supervisor' and 'supervisee' as both are consistent with a biomedical approach (*see* List 10.1) and an external locus of control (*see* Explanation box 10.4). For example, the words 'supervisor' and 'supervisee' infer:

Supervisor:	Supervisee:
Manager	Underling
Administrator	Recipient
Superintendent	Minion
Controller	Inferior
Overseer	Junior
Director	Subordinate
Boss	Assistant
Superior	Follower

The words 'supervisor' and 'supervisee' can lead to negative interpretations of a process that is in no way consistent with person-centred development. As such, we need to find new words to replace supervisor and supervisee. I offer the words 'facilitator' and 'participant' because both words are consistent with a biopsychosocial approach and an internal locus of control (*see* Explanation box 10.4). They infer:

Facilitator:	Participant:
Enhance	To make a choice
Helper	To contribute
Support	To be a part of
Development	To protect
Assist	To be sincere
Improve	To be honest
Kind	To care
Compassionate	To reflect and develop

As can be seen from the above, facilitator and participant are consistent with

Bond and Holland's (1998) definition and that person-centred development should be a process that is about people and caring. Therefore, from this point on I shall apply the words 'facilitator' and 'participant' in place of 'supervisor' and 'supervisee'.

To continue our discussion on models, there are some models in existence that are reflective of person-centred development and as such have the potential to facilitate greater levels of adherence to standard precautions if appropriately applied by an astute facilitator. Such models include the biopsychosocial approach (*see* List 10.2), the development model (Leddick 1994), the friendship model (Smith 2000) and Maslow's Hierarchy of Needs (Potter and Perry 2001). In considering each of these models, let's begin with the biopsychosocial approach (*see* List 10.2).

REFLECTION EXERCISE 10.6

What do you feel is positive about the biopsychosocial approach where person-centred development is concerned?

If you were facilitating a person-centred development session, what physical, psychological and social factors might have an effect upon the session?

If you were receiving person-centred development, what physical, psychological or social factors might affect your feelings about the session?

For facilitators to effectively apply this approach they must have an understanding that within a person-centred development session, physical, psychological and social factors will always be present and will impact upon the facilitator and the participant(s) (*see* List 10.4).

LIST 10.4 PHYSICAL, PSYCHOLOGICAL AND SOCIAL FACTORS IMPACTING UPON PERSON-CENTRED DEVELOPMENT SESSIONS (ELLIOTT CITED IN JASPER 2006; ROPER, LOGAN AND TIERNEY 2000)

Physical factors:
1 Environmental – heating, lighting, temperature, available space, equipment, ventilation.
2 Work load.
3 Body clock – day duty, night duty.
4 Levels of stress and fatigue.
5 Comfort – whether rest breaks are taken, fluid balance, nutritional state, elimination when necessary.

6   Play – inclusion of humour, laughter, smiling, tone of voice.

Psychological factors:
1   Levels of stress and anxiety.
2   Mood and emotional state.
3   Past experiences of person-centred development.
4   Was the facilitator chosen or given?
5   Feeling safe and secure.
6   Communication –
    Verbal:
    ● What is said.
    ● How something is said.
    ● Language/jargon used.

    Non-verbal:
    ● Facial expression.
    ● Posture.
    ● Style of dress.
    ● Smiling.

    Written:
    ● Covert or open making of notes.
    ● Who can access notes made.
    ● Setting of ground rules.

Social factors:
1   Drawing up ground rules.
2   Relationship – facilitative or dictatorial.
3   Freedom of expression.
4   Locus of control – internal or external.
5   Play – positive interactions, humour and laughter.
6   Confidentiality – ground rules (what is discussed).

NB: The above should not be seen as being mutually exclusive but as offering examples.

For example, the physical environment will impact upon how receptive a participant is towards reflecting upon their adherence to standard precautions. If the area being used for the session is not comfortable (e.g. temperature is too high or too low), is too public and subject to interruptions, then these will impact upon all the participants' sense of comfort and security. As a result, their focus will be orientated towards whether they feel too hot or cold and whether what they say will be overheard by others. Subsequently, the degree to which a participant will be willing to reflect upon their adherence to standard precautions will be negligible. This is because they will be orientated towards self-preservation, concerned that if they discuss their failings regarding standard precautions and others outside of the confidential setting hear what they say, this may have consequences for them. Therefore careful consideration should be give to the environment within which person-centred development occurs.

Psychological factors can have a powerful impact upon the degree to which a participant will openly discuss and reflect upon their adherence to standard precautions. For example, suppose the participant's facilitator is also their line manager. In such a situation there exists a conflict of interest for the facilitator/ manager in that what is discussed and reflected upon within a confidential person-centred development session may require the facilitator, in their management role, to instigate disciplinary action against the participant. Within such a context there are clearly professional, ethical, moral and human rights issues. Such a situation will be likely to cause a participant to feel anxious and stressed about honestly discussing their level of adherence to standard precautions. Yet that situation, where facilitators and managers are the same person, occurs all too frequently within health and social care. For example, some health and social care professionals not only find the term 'clinical supervision' acceptable, but also instigate it from a biomedical perspective, use it as a means of monitoring standards and see it as being perfectly acceptable to allocate potential participants to individuals they consider will make good supervisors with no consultation with the potential participant concerned. The ethics of such an approach is highly questionable. However, perhaps those health or social care professionals who choose to adopt such an approach care little for the ethics of what they do (Seedhouse 1998).

REFLECTION EXERCISE 10.7

How do you feel about the idea that many health and social care professionals may care little for the ethics of what they do?

You may want to reflect upon this from two perspectives:

1   If you have in the past or are currently undertaking person-centred development (clinical supervision) how was your facilitator (supervisor) selected? Were you able or allowed to make the choice or was that person chosen for you?

If that person was chosen for you, were your feelings taken into account? If not, and you were simply told that this person would be your supervisor, how much do you feel the ethics of such a decision were considered?

2   Think about how well you adhere to standard precautions. Can you in absolute honesty state that you have always adopted standard precautions appropriately and when you knew you should?

Current healthcare-acquired infection rates are thought to be primarily due to health and social care professionals' failures to adopt appropriate infection-control practices (e.g. standard precautions) (Stone *et al.* 2004). In the past, if you have failed to wash your hands properly, for example, what are the ethical implications of that? How much consideration have you given to the ethics of what you have not done?

At this point ask yourself these questions:

How guilty and uncomfortable do I feel about the ethics of my actions or acts of omission?

How guilty and uncomfortable should I be feeling?

Perhaps some health and social care professionals are more concerned about using person-centred development sessions as a means of fostering a blaming culture. Such an approach will fail to have any impact upon non-adherence to standard precautions and will be more likely to indirectly increase such non-adherence.

REFLECTION EXERCISE 10.8

In reflecting upon the reasons why some health and social care professionals instigate person-centred development as a means of finding fault and applying blame, why might this cause an increase in non-adherence to standard precautions?

In undertaking this exercise, you may wish to reflect on your conclusions from Reflection exercise 10.7.

The idea of person-centred development is to facilitate individuals in thinking about where they may have failed to adequately adhere to standard precautions. However, where person-centred development is used to find fault, to foster a blaming culture and as a tool for managing, controlling or monitoring, it is likely that participants' stress and anxiety levels will increase. As a result, they will choose not to reflect upon and discuss their adoption of standard precautions. Therefore, how a facilitator is chosen and by whom, and who that facilitator is, must be given careful consideration. Get it wrong and non-adherence to standard precautions will likely not change and may increase. Get it right and the potential for reducing non-adherence to standard precautions will be enhanced.

Social factors can also impact upon the extent to which a participant interacts within a person-centred development session. Many within health and social care perceive person-centred development to be unidirectional; for example, facilitator to participant. Such an approach within any social setting will negatively impact upon the quality of interaction that occurs. Therefore, an exchange of reflective thoughts and ideas will be restricted, if not prevented, from occurring. Interaction is a vital aspect of the person-centred development process and must always be multidirectional.

All those present within the session must be accepted as equal and be permitted to express themselves. Failure to do this will constitute an infringement of a participant's human rights (*see* List 10.3). The idea that the facilitator is not there to gain from the experience and that person-centred development sessions are only about facilitating the personal and professional development of the participant(s) is in itself dissonance-based and cognitively economic thinking (*see* Explanation boxes 10.1 and 10.2).

Person-centred development is for everyone and within this context the role of facilitator and participant should be interchangeable (Elliott cited in Jasper 2006). The philosophy that should be adopted is that the process will always be multidirectional and the social interaction that occurs is vital to the success of person-centred development. A multidirectional approach within a trusting and confidential setting will facilitate differing perspectives and promote the right of all to express their feelings and opinions, because talking and listening will serve to facilitate reflective thought and raise awareness. If the physical, psychological and social factors are recognised and taken into account, the potential for person-centred development to reduce non-adherence to standard precautions will be increased.

Developmental model

The developmental (Leddick 1994) model is consistent with the philosophies set out within a biopsychosocial approach (*see* List 10.2). The developmental model can also be linked with the concept of lifelong learning, as it sees individuals as continually growing and developing. This is, of course, fundamental to the idea of person-centred development. For example, after the facilitator and participant have set ground rules during the first session, the process is an ongoing one. However, this should not necessitate the need to structure or set predetermined agendas. Rather, the process should be allowed to flow naturally. Within a person-centred development session, reflecting upon past experiences can be used to facilitate the future actions of those taking part. These experiences can then be investigated in greater depth regarding their cause and evaluated. For example, a participant or facilitator might attempt to explain the reason for their past non-adherence to standard precautions, which resulted from their not having enough time to meet their patients' or clients' needs if they followed the hand hygiene process exactly (*see* List 10.5). In reflecting on this the aim would be to increase their awareness and understanding that failing to follow the hand hygiene process would not be consistent with meeting patients' or clients' needs.

LIST 10.5 HAND HYGIENE PROCESS (ELLIOTT 2003)

Stage 1 – It is vital that you recognise the need to undertake hand hygiene. This is probably the most important stage within the process because if you fail to recognise situations where you need to adopt formal hand hygiene, as opposed to using cleansing gels, then the remainder of the process will at worst not occur and at best occur intermittently. Either way the risk of cross infection will be increased.

Stage 2 – It is important that you wet all areas to be washed thoroughly with running water. Failure do this may lead to you experiencing skin problems because some cleansing agents can cause irritation of the skin if applied prior to wetting the areas to be washed. The rule being always read the manufacturer's recommendations.

Stage 3 – It is important that you always apply an appropriate cleansing agent to the areas for washing. They type of agent will be determined by the nature of the intended intervention:
- invasive/surgical
- antiseptic
- social.

It is not necessary to apply excessive amounts of the cleansing solution and the manufacturer's recommendations should always be followed.

Stage 4 – It is important that you use running water when washing the areas of your body to be cleansed/decontaminated, using an approved method and time period:
- invasive/surgical: minimum 2 minutes – hands, wrists and up to the elbow;

- antiseptic: minimum 30 seconds – hands, wrists and up to mid-forearm;
- social: minimum 15 seconds – hands and wrists.

Stage 5 – It is important that you rinse all the areas washed, until all trace of the cleansing agent has gone. Failure to do this may lead to skin irritation resulting from traces of the cleansing agent being left on your skin. In addition, where traces of the cleansing agent are left on the skin this may serve to facilitate bacterial re-colonisation.

Stage 6 – It is important to thoroughly dry all of the areas washed, using:
- sterile hand towels for invasive/surgical interventions;
- sterile or disposable hand towels depending upon the nature of the intervention antiseptic to be used;
- disposable hand towels or hot air blowers for social interventions.

Friendship model

The friendship model (Smith 2000) is also consistent with a biopsychosocial approach (*see* List 10.2) and the concept of lifelong learning. The idea of friendship can equate to the development of a trusting relationship. Within the context of successful person-centred development where all involved are to grow, develop and benefit, trust must exist. Without trust, honesty will be lacking and if person-centred development is to improve adherence to standard precautions then all involved must feel they can be open and honest with each other. Trust and honesty can be facilitated if:
➤ the participant is allowed to choose their facilitator;
➤ the facilitator is not their manager;
➤ it is generally recognised that a participant's facilitator does not have to be of the same profession or even work within the same department or organisation;
➤ ground rules are set and agreed by all involved;
➤ any notes that are taken are given to all involved;
➤ all those involved feel comfortable and relaxed through the presence of:
  — humour
  — language used
  — tone of voice
  — open and non-threatening body language
  — an appropriate environment is found
  — temperature, lighting and seating are comfortable.
➤ a recognition that roles within person-centred development sessions may be interchangeable: facilitator becomes participant and vice versa.

Friendship within the context of trust and honesty are crucial elements of the person-centred development process. If these elements are not present, an individual's non-adherence to standard precautions is more likely because a participant will not reflect upon their failings. Rather, they will tend to adopt a defensive stance reinforced by dissonance-based excuses (*see* Explanation box 10.1) and cognitively economic perspectives (*see* Explanation box 10.2). As a consequence they will have little, if any, impact upon reducing non-adherence to standard precautions.

Maslow's hierachy of needs

Finally, let's consider Maslow's hierarchy of needs (Potter and Perry 2001) as a facilitator for improving adherence to standard precautions within a person-centred development context. All individuals taking part in a person-centred development session will bring with them specific needs. During the course of a session those needs will be in constant flux. Within his hierarchy Maslow proposed five levels of need (*see* Figure 10.3).

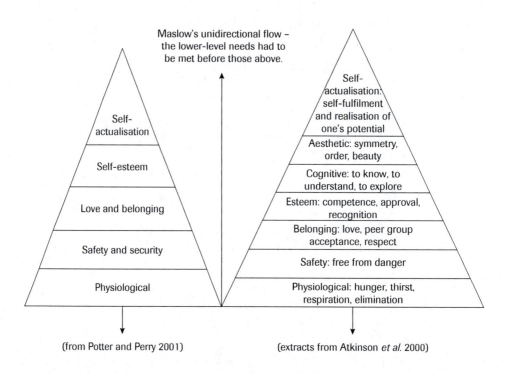

FIGURE 10.3 Maslow's hierarchy of needs. Adapted from Atkinson RL *et al. Hilgard's Introduction to Psychology.* 13th ed. London: International Thomson Publishing; 2000.

It is important that a facilitator of person-centred development has an awareness of the participants' needs, their complexity and the impact they can have upon the quality and outcome of a person-centred development session. For example, if a participant arrives at a session having not taken adequate nutrition or fluids, then it is likely that their blood sugar will be affected. That, in turn, will impact upon their cognitive functioning, which may lead to misinterpretation and misunderstanding resulting in, for example, a sense of insecurity. A facilitator must be alert to such situations if all involved are to get the best out of a session. The essence of using Maslow's hierarchy as a model for facilitating person-centred development is in providing an understanding that if a recipient's needs are not accounted for, recognised and supported, personal and professional growth and development will be affected.

It is crucial that a facilitator tries to ensure that the needs of all participants are met when necessary; for example, prior to a session commencing a facilitator should prepare the environment so that the seating is comfortable, tea, coffee and water are available and, most importantly, greet the participant(s) with a smile. A smile is a wonderful thing and has a positive psychological effect. Ensuring that these sorts of things occur will serve to facilitate to a recipient's physiological, safety, belongingness and esteem needs (*see* Figure 10.3). Cognitive needs can be facilitated through, for example, the style and methods of communication used: open body posture, a smile, eye contact and tone of voice. Aesthetic and self-actualisation needs can be facilitated over time and can be related to the establishment of trust and everyone involved gaining a sense of achievement from the sessions.

However, if Maslow's hierarchy is to be used as a model to facilitate person-centred development there is a need to re-define the hierarchy's initial premise. Maslow proposed that individuals could only meet each of the needs in a unidirectional way, going from the base of the triangle to the top. However, this premise is flawed (Elliott 1992).

REFLECTION EXERCISE 10.9

In looking at Figure 10.3 can you think of any reasons why this unidirectional premise was established, that each need has to be met in a unidirectional way?

In undertaking Reflection exercise 10.9, you may have determined that none of these needs actually occur in such a logical sequence. In fact, to accept such a unidirectional sequence as being logical is dissonance-based (*see* Explanation

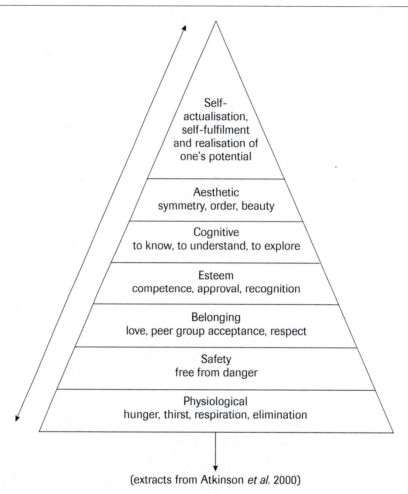

(extracts from Atkinson *et al.* 2000)

FIGURE 10.4 Re-evaluating Maslow's hierarchy of needs. Adapted from Atkinson RL *et al. Hilgard's Introduction to Psychology.* 13th ed. London: International Thomson Publishing; 2000.

box 10.1) and cognitively economic (*see* Explanation box 10.2). Rather, they are in constant flux. Our needs are prioritised depending upon how we feel, for example, where we are and what we have been doing or wish to do. In reality, we meet the needs set out within Maslow's hierarchy on a continuum basis (Elliott 1992) (*see* Figure 10.4).

When applying Maslow's hierarchy to a facilitator of person-centred development, it must be viewed as a two-directional continuum where needs are prioritised as they arise and not in a unidirectional way from the base of the triangle upwards (Elliott 1992). With regards to self-actualisation, this should be achievable on a rolling basis. For example, being praised for a particular behaviour or passing a test may cause the individual to feel a sense of self-fulfilment and of having achieved their potential in a given thing.

To assume that an individual's physical/physiological needs have to be met first is reflective of dissonance-based thinking (*see* Explanation box 10.1) and a cognitively economic perspective (*see* Explanation box 10.2). Human needs are in constant flux and an individual will give priority to the need that imposes the greatest influence at any given time. For example, the need to feel safe may override the individual's need for food. However, an individual's need to explore (curiosity) may override safety needs.

According to a unidirectional approach (*see* Figure 10.3), if we are hungry but have to cross a busy road to get to the food store, our physiological needs would have to be met before we could meet any of our other needs. As such we would step out into the road without looking or considering our safety and may get knocked down by a motor vehicle. However, in general we tend not do this. Although we may be hungry, in order to satisfy that need our safety

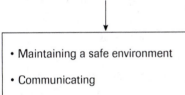

Activities of living

- Maintaining a safe environment
- Communicating
- Breathing
- Eating and drinking
- Eliminating
- Personal cleansing and dressing
- Controlling body temperature
- Mobilising
- Working
- Playing
- Expressing sexuality
- Sleeping
- Dying

Achieving each of these involves physical activity across the life span. If an individual becomes unable to carry out one or more of these activities they will experience physical, psychological and social consequences.

For example:

- An inability to mobilise will prevent or restrict an individual's ability to get from one place to another.

- An inability to maintain a safe environment will result in stress and anxiety being experienced.

- An inability to play (bearing in mind that adults play as much as children, just in a different way) could result in social isolation.

FIGURE 10.5 Activities of daily living.

takes priority, thus allowing us to cross the busy road safely so we can satisfy our physiological need to eat.

What is interesting is that being able to prioritise in this way is a consequence of both nature and nurture. One might argue that a unidirectional progression of meeting needs might exist for young children. For example, a young child would simply know that they were hungry and forget to ensure it was safe to cross the road. This presents us with a nature perspective on Maslow's hierarchy. However, as we grow older, we learn from others about the dangers inherent in crossing the road. We do this partly through what we are told by our parents and significant others (a nurture perspective) and partly through mirror neurons (Dobbs 2006), which are physiological structures that enable each of us to innately copy the behaviour of others.

Therefore, Maslow's hierarchy can be viewed from both nature and nurture perspectives. As we grow, we learn to prioritise the order in which we meet our needs and activities of daily living (*see* Figure 10.5). In placing this within a person-centred development context, a facilitator must have an awareness of this ability to prioritise needs and apply Maslow's hierarchy in a flexible manner (*see* Figure 10.4). To apply the hierarchy in a unidirectional manner will potentially lead to needs not adequately being met. If a participant's needs are not recognised and met, this will disrupt the session and, in turn, fail to promote the safe adoption of standard precautions. This is because the recipient will be more focused on meeting their needs as opposed to reflecting upon their adoption of standard precautions. Therefore, Maslow's hierarchy can be used to promote the reduction of non-adherence to standard precautions.

Before concluding this chapter I would like to return to the idea of eye contact which is an important aspect in the establishment of a positive person-centred development relationship. If too much eye contact is made then it can be interpreted by an individual as aggressive intimidation leading to the individual feeling uneasy, stressed and anxious. On the other hand too little eye contact can be interpreted as disinterest, lack of caring or being bored. Whether it be too much or too little eye contact, both will have a negative effect upon a person-centred development relationship.

Eye contact is a skilled activity and involves, for example, an understanding of positioning and where to look when not making eye contact. For example, in a one-to-one person-centred development session the ideal positioning is a 45-degree angle to each other whilst taking into account body spacing. Thus when eye contact is not being made there is a visual escape route to look away from the other person. The problem arises when such a visual escape route does not exist. For example, if the individuals are positioned facing or opposite each other where do you look when not making eye contact?

If you are facing or directly opposite another individual where do you look when not making eye contact?

With regards to the responses you gave to Reflection exercise 10.10 you might have identified:

➤ Looking to the left or right.
➤ Looking down.
➤ Looking up.

The problem is that in carrying out any of these three actions above your eyes may only move a matter of millimetres. Therefore if you look to the left or right of the individuals face it may appear to them that you are still making eye contact (looking at them), which may be interpreted as staring. If you look down the individual may interpret this as you looking at other parts of their body or being condescending, which could have anxiety provoking effects. If you look up with your eyes this could be interpreted as patronising, dismissive, condescending or that you are simply not interested.

Eye contact is a vital aspect of any interpersonal relationship and as such is highly relevant to person-centred development context. Get eye contact right and it can have a positive impact. Get it wrong and it can be very destructive to the relationship.

CONCLUSION

There can be no doubt that person-centred development can play a part in helping to reduce non-adherence to standard precautions. However, in order to make this process more effective, we need to change the current term 'clinical supervision' to 'person-centred development' and ensure that appropriate models are applied. In addition, we need to move away from the titles of 'supervisor' and 'supervisee' as these are both consistent with a biomedical approach (*see* List 10.1). More appropriate terms are 'facilitator' (someone who supports) and 'participant(s)' (one or more people who choose to undertake person-centred development). There is no reason why several models could not be applied. For example, combining a biopsychosocial approach (*see* List 10.2), the friendship model (Smith 2000) and Maslow's hierarchy (*see* Figure 10.4) would serve to provide a number of sources from which to offer person-centred development.

REFERENCES

Adams B, Bromley B. *Psychology for Healthcare: key terms and concepts.* London: Macmillan; 1998.

Atkinson RL, Atkinson RC, Smith E, *et al. Hilgard's Introduction to Psychology.* 13th ed. London: Harcourt College Publishers; 2000.

Bond M, Holland S. *Skills of Clinical Supervision for Nurses: a practical guide for supervisees, clinical supervisors and managers.* Buckingham: Open University Press; 1998.

Dobbs D. A revealing reflection. *Sci Am Mind.* 2006; **17**: 22–7.

Elliott P. Handwashing: a process of judgement and effective decision making. *Prof Nurse.* 1992; **7**(5): 292–6.

Elliott P. Recognising the psychosocial issues involved in hand hygiene. *J R Soc Promo Health.* 2003; **123**(2): 88–94.

Elliott P. Understanding clinical supervision: a health psychology orientated process of person-centred development. In: Jasper M, editor. *Vital Notes for Nurses: professional development, reflection and decision making.* Oxford: Blackwell Publishing; 2006.

Engle G. Personal theories of disease as determinants of patient-physician relationships. In: Skevington S. *Psychology of Pain.* Chichester: John Wiley; 1996.

Festinger L. Cognitive dissonance. *Sci Am.* 1962; **207**: 93–102.

Howatson-Jones IL. Difficulties in clinical supervision and lifelong learning. *Nurs Stand.* 2003; **17**(37): 37–41.

Leddick G. Models of clinical supervision. 1994. *ERIC Digest.* Available at: http://ericdigests.org/1995-1/models.htm (accessed 25 Nov 2008).

Ogden J. *Health Psychology: a textbook.* 4th ed. Maidenhead: Open University Press/McGraw-Hill; 2007.

Potter P, Perry A. *Fundamentals of Nursing.* 5th ed. London: Mosby; 2001.

Roper N, Logan W, Tierney A. *The Roper-Logan-Tierney Model of Nursing: based on activities of living.* London: Churchill Livingstone; 2000.

Roth I, Frisby J. *Perception and Representation: a cognitive approach.* Milton Keynes: Open University; 1992.

Seedhouse D. *Ethics: the heart of healthcare.* Chichester: John Wiley and Sons; 1998.

Sloan G, Watson H. Clinical supervision models for nursing: structure, research and limitations. *Nurs Stand.* 2002; **17**(4): 41–6.

Smith G. Friendship within clinical supervision: a model for the NHS. Presentation for launch of *National Nursing Strategy for Wales: realising the potential.* Sept 2000.

Stone P, Clarke S, Cimiotti J, Correa-de-Araujo R. Nurses' working conditions: implications for infectious disease. *Emerg Infect Dis* (International Conference on Women and Infectious Diseases). 2004; **10**(11): 1984–9.

Wallston K, Wallston B. Who is responsible for your health?: the construct of health locus of control. In: Sanders G, Suls J, editors. *Social Psychology of Health and Illness.* Hillsdale: Erlbaum; 1982.

Wilkinson R, Caulfield H. *The Human Rights Act: a practical guide for nurses.* Chichester: John Wiley; 2001.

INTRODUCTION

Sue Clark and I have known each other as colleagues for several years within the Department of Nursing and Applied Clinical Studies at Canterbury Christ Church University. As colleagues, we have worked together on a number of occasions and in that time I have developed a healthy respect for her ability to apply the concepts that underpin adult learning to the real world of infection management. Sue's expertise within this area is well-recognised. As you read through her chapter, you may find it useful to reflect upon its potential within your workplace.

CHAPTER 11

Facilitating infection-control practice through education: is this the only way?

Sue Clark

This chapter aims to explore how infection control education has been delivered in the past and will question those approaches in the light of significant advances in access to information. Changes in management of the NHS and working practices, developments in surgical techniques and device use, an aging population, increased use of antimicrobial agents, and as Pittet (2005) noted, the shortening of patient hospital stays leading to an aggregation of sicker patients, have all had an impact on the prevention and control of infection. The challenge now is to look at new approaches to information provision and involve the psychosocial aspects that impact on behaviour in an effort to improve the patient experience of healthcare.

In order to address a range of approaches to learning and behaviour change, it is necessary to review the multimodal approaches from the behavioural sciences, such as motivation, intention, perception of threat and outcomes expectancy as part of the learning experience, as well as the concept of social marketing, and institutional policy and sanctions (Mah, Deshpande and Rothschild 2006; Pittet 2005).

Patient expectations have increased (Department of Health [DoH] 2000) and it seems that patients who acquire infection that leads to morbidity or loss of life are now more likely to seek redress through the courts, substantially increasing costs to the NHS (McIntosh 2005). Media interest in infection issues has also risen and although it may have helped to fuel increases in litigation, the publicity surrounding poor practices should also be the stimulus for improvement. There is considerable evidence to indicate that healthcare-associated infection is a major problem (National Audit Office [NAO] 2000; NAO 2004; Sheng *et al.* 2005) but improvements are slow. The Office for National Statistics indicated that in one region, deaths from *C. difficile* had trebled (BBC 2007) and there is a suggestion that MRSA superbug claims may surge as lawyers are making use of the laws governing the control of hazardous substances (BBC 2006). To improve public confidence and patient safety, it is paramount that each healthcare worker recognises their professional responsibility in the safe delivery of care and treatment to reduce the risk of infection both within the acute and community sectors.

Duckworth (2003) noted that although MRSA is predominantly acquired in hospital, reports of community-acquired MRSA was a worrying development and although the causative strains often differed from hospital ones, it still posed a big challenge for control and treatment within units such as care homes and prisons. This challenge must include provision of updates to all heathcare workers in all settings and this must be facilitated through robust communication mechanisms and strong leadership.

Education is generally acknowledged as an act or process of developing knowledge and skills, and evidence of the ability to learn is required before entering a professional occupation. In the healthcare professions, continuous professional development is necessary to maintain professional registration (BMA 2005; HPC 2005; Nursing and Midwifery Council [NMC] 2006) and this means that learning becomes lifelong. This helps to ensure that research is identified and acted upon to provide the best evidence base for practice. However, the acquisition of knowledge without a change in behaviour is considered by Bloom (1956) to be of the lower order of learning and does not demonstrate an ability to comprehend or understand the concepts and apply and evaluate the learning. It is suggested that this element is crucial in the healthcare setting where change in practice behaviour is evidence of the application of knowledge.

REFLECTION EXERCISE 11.1

Consider the last occasion that you increased your knowledge and understanding of an infection control-related issue.

Who or what were the means of that learning?

Facilitating safe infection-control practice through education has always been one of the core functions of infection-control activity (DoH 1995; Haley, Culver and White 1985; Jenner and Wilson 2000; King 2005). This aimed to provide people with information about how infection was spread, how it could be prevented and how it could be managed (Chalmers and Straub 2006; McCulloch 1998). The implied outcome was that healthcare workers would modify their behaviour as a result of their education and increased awareness of the risks to patients. Mah, Deshpande and Rothschild (2006) noted that the educational approach was usually supported by an infection control policy produced by the infection control team (ICT).

Experience of infection-control education in the 1970s and 80s as a ward nurse involved a short talk from an infection control nurse (ICN) on hand hygiene and little else. Often this was ward-based and there were limitations to this approach in that it tended to be didactic in style with little learner involvement. As shift patterns and work practices changed, fewer staff attended these sessions so the emergence of the role of link nurse provided a source of information for others. They were developed in their role through short courses and regular updates to enable them to share good practice (Horton 1988) and be a link with the ICT. There was a concern about link nurses though, that other staff might view them as being responsible for infection control, thereby potentially absolving individuals from personal responsibility for their actions.

The literature indicates that even in the late 1970s, only 64% of health districts had appointed an ICN and only 18% of those had any specialist education (Perry 2005). It was noted that one ICN had responsibility, on average, for 741 beds (Knappett 1981), which may have accounted for the limited educational input. The speciality gained a higher profile after an outbreak of salmonella at the Stanley Royd Hospital in Wakefield and the DHSS (1988) issued the first guidance document on hospital infection control, which required on ICN in each health district who had received post-basic education. However, it was interesting to note that even though ICN numbers increased, they had, on average, responsibility for 853 beds and this was probably because mental health settings were now included.

The 1990s experienced a decade of change and development as well as difficulties, and included NHS reorganisation, mounting problems with MRSA, the move of nurse education into universities, increases in litigation, and development of clinical governance standards and risk management. Demands by the DoH for more information on aspects of infection within hospitals and increases in ICT personnel were required to carry out surveillance activities to meet the requirements for information through the Nosocomial Infection National Surveillance Scheme. The role of education was even more important, and how best to incorporate it became even more of a challenge.

The Professional Codes of Conduct require healthcare workers to act always in the interests of patients and clients and minimise risks (NMC 2004, 2008) and protect and promote health of patients (GMC 2006). Staff are also required to work within the Health and Safety at Work Act regulations and Control of Substances Hazardous to Health, which includes micro-organisms and body fluids. Failure to address appropriate hand hygiene practices could be seen as a breach of the professional code of conduct, and as patients become more aware of good practice this could be an issue which they pursue if affected by infection.

REFLECTION EXERCISE 11.2

What factors do you consider when making a decision on whether or not to decontaminate your hands?

Have there been occasions when you have not performed hand hygiene and can you recall why this happened?

Do you consider that you have an ethical/moral obligation to reduce the risk of infection to those in your care?

Do you believe that hand hygiene has a role to play in infection prevention?

The evidence shows that care is compromised in specific areas of practice and includes hand hygiene (Boyce 1999; Huggonet, Perneger and Pittet 2002; Pittet *et al.* 2000,), and barrier precautions (Larsen and Kretzer 1995) – two of the core procedures probably most associated with good practice. Reasons suggested for non-compliance have included heavy work loads, glove use and technical procedures and facilities (Karabey *et al.* 2002; Naikoba and Hayward 2001; Osbourne 2003). The evidence base for the effectiveness of hand hygiene in patient care is indisputable and highlights reduced rates of infection when performed correctly (Larsen *et al.* 2000; Pittet *et al.* 2000; MacDonald *et al.* 2004; Sud and Gorman 2007).

Evidence for the use of barrier precautions such as gloves and aprons is also well-acknowledged (Pellowe *et al.* 2004; UK Health Dept 1998). However, as Karabey *et al.* (2002) noted, this lack of compliance with these procedures is likely to be part of a bigger picture where many staff fail to adhere to recommended infection-control behaviour.

The DoH (2003, 2004, 2005, 2006) has consistently been concerned about poor infection-control practices and produced new documents, standards and mandatory training to address this, but there remains concern about levels of healthcare-associated infection. Are there other factors apart from the educational issues that need to be considered?

It has been suggested that the culture of an organisation can have an impact on behaviour within the workplace in relation to change (Senge *et al.* 1999). The 'culture' of a group can indicate to others the way things are done or generally the values that are important to it. Senge *et al.* (1999) suggests that there is a fundamental flaw in most change strategies because they focus on the change rather than understanding how the culture will react to their efforts. The NHS culture is likely to vary from one location to another, but Wilson and Greaves (2002) note that in professional organisations, people like to be independent and follow their own judgement and will listen to peers and experts, but are reluctant to take orders from management. The delivery programme on Saving Lives (DoH 2006) may demonstrate clear reductions in HCAI because it has identified the need to have ownership of change, which leads to cooperation and an appreciation of personal responsibility as well as engagement, which is critical to success. The NHS, as other care organisations, involves people both as patients and staff, and attention must be given to people-management skills if progress is to occur.

REFLECTION EXERCISE 11.3

How would you describe the culture of your work environment?

If it is a ward who leads on infection issues?

Are there role models and is it supportive on infection control issues?

How would you feel and react if challenged by a patient who had seen you perform care of another patient and then you attend to their needs without decontamination of your hands?

If you work as a nurse in the community setting, who provides leadership on infection-control issues and are there updates available?

If you are a practice nurse, when did you last receive an infection-control update and from whom?

If you had concerns about decontamination issues, with whom would you discuss these problems?

It can be helpful to review examples of improvements in practice and tease out the factors that contributed to their success. A study by Pittet *et al.* (2000) demonstrated clear improvements in hand hygiene practices by implementing a hospital-wide programme with emphasis on bedside alcohol-based hand decontamination. This study involved seven observational surveys between

1994 and 1997, and demonstrated improvements in hand hygiene from 48% at the start to 66% at the end of the study. The secondary outcome measure was a decrease in nosocomial infection from 16.9% at the start to 9.9% at the finish.

Another example was the National Patient Safety Agency (NPSA) Clean Your Hands campaign, which also used near-patient alcohol rubs as part of its strategy (Randle, Clarke and Storr 2006). Six acute Trusts in England were included and it was described as a multimodal campaign and included alcohol hand rubs, posters, marketing materials, such as badges, and leaflets for patients encouraging them to ask staff about hand hygiene. After six months, the results indicated a marked increase in hand hygiene from 32% at the start to 63% at the finish and the majority of patients indicated that the public should be actively involved in helping healthcare workers to improve hand hygiene. However, the literature suggested that the 16 respondents who answered questions on asking staff about hand hygiene generally did not feel comfortable with this aspect, although they considered that the campaign made them feel more confident.

The components in the success of the first study by Pittet *et al.* (2000) included a multidisciplinary project team with senior managers as well as representatives from every hospital department. Involvement of senior management and their regular attendance at meetings indicated a high level of commitment to the project. Over 70 different coloured posters were produced (some using cartoons), and displayed in strategic positions in the hospital and changed each week. Jenner *et al.* (2005) noted that the most effective health promotion behaviour should be framed in terms of gains rather than losses, or positive rather than negative language. The availability of alcohol rubs at the bedside, as well as individual alcohol bottles, facilitated hand hygiene practices and performance feedback was undertaken with results in hospital newsletters. As this was a multi-strategy project, it was difficult to determine which intervention was the most vital in its success, but the authors attributed it mainly to the alcohol hand rubs.

The second study also used bedside alcohol rubs, and posters with the addition of marketing materials, such as badges. One difference was that patients were provided with leaflets that encouraged them to ask staff about their hand hygiene. The Department of Health (NHS Plan 2000) promoted patient empowerment and two studies (McGuckin 1999, 2001) aimed to work with patients to improve staff hand hygiene and it indicated that patients can be empowered to be responsible for reducing risks in self-care. However, there are concerns that not all patients can or want to become involved and as Williams (2002) noted, outcomes in relation to patient empowerment are not well-documented; neither is the impact on staff. As the Randle, Clarke and Storr (2006) study observed, patients were not always comfortable with asking staff about hand hygiene. Williams (2002) suggested that staff empowerment is a critical antecedent to patient empowerment and it seems fitting that, as healthcare workers, the delivery of safe care is an integral component of professional responsibility.

REFLECTION EXERCISE 11.4

What factors in your workplace do you consider may make it more likely that you compromise best clinical practice?

Consider how these might be addressed and who might be involved.

Probably one of the biggest challenges today is the delivery of appropriate, relevant and research-based education that encourages and motivates staff to want to comply with recommended practices so that infections are reduced. It is worth looking at current approaches to learn about infection prevention and control before reviewing the behavioural aspects that are so critical in achieving compliance.

Information is freely available over the Internet regarding most aspects of life, but obviously it is essential to obtain robust information around professional practice from reliable sources where research is included. These can be books, journals, or online packages provided through a professional body or employing organisation. Websites such as the Department of Health (DoH) or Health Protection Agency (HPA) sites also provide information both to the public and healthcare workers. Most employers – especially the NHS – now have policies in hard copy as well as available online for reference. Opportunities for self-development include not only e-learning, but blended learning, which combines two or more approaches. However, Walsh (2005) noted the technology must be tailored to meet the outcomes so that communication skills, for example, are not only addressed through e-learning, but face-to-face encounters. In healthcare, three areas are considered important for development and include knowledge, skills and attitudes (NMC 2004) and it seems appropriate that assessment of the latter two will involve face-to-face contact. Regardless, there are few learning technologies that can compete with an enthusiastic, knowledgeable, expert. Study days, short courses, lectures and seminars are important ways of engaging with a subject and developing knowledge and understanding, and must not be relegated because of technological progress.

How do you learn and what or who provided your most inspirational learning experience?

An understanding of how people learn is important if knowledge is to be integrated into behavioural change. There has been a considerable shift away from the didactic approach to learning where students were passive recipients of information, towards a more interactive style where students are actively involved in their learning. Dewey (1963) was an early proponent of 'progressive' education. He recognised that educators needed to be aware of the whole learner experience and that it was likely to be connected to personal experience as well as previous learning. He realised that the connection to wider and deeper experiences would be critical in the integration of subsequent learning. Development of work-based learning packages has helped to encourage students to use reflection on their prior knowledge and experience, and link it to formal knowledge and practice; thereby increasing their overall learning (Gallaher and Holland 2004).

One of the major difficulties with infection control learning is that it does not always seem to translate into behaviour change, especially around decontamination of hands. Cole (2006) suggests that although hand hygiene is a simple act, it is carried out within a complex organisational system and therefore interventions to improve compliance must reflect these complexities. Storr and Clayton-Kent (2004) suggest a range of strategies, such as education, role modelling, management support, observation and feedback, posters, and publication of infection rates, but recognise that there is no single strategy that achieves improvements in compliance.

Cole (2006) briefly explores a range of learning theories, such as behaviourism, cognitivism, role modelling, and motivational theory, but reaches the conclusion that individual motivation and behaviour are extremely sophisticated concepts and cannot always be manipulated or enhanced by traditional approaches to education. However, it is worth noting that studies that have used a range of approaches have demonstrated sustained improvements in hand hygiene.

In a study of patients in a plastic surgery unit by MacDonald *et al.* (2004), the numbers of new patients acquiring MRSA were halved after the introduction of feedback on hand hygiene performance. A study by Rao *et al.* (2002) used many of the precepts of social marketing, which included a premarketing analysis of strengths, weaknesses, opportunities and threats (SWOT) to improvements in hand hygiene and a review of products and prices, promotion issues and accessibility of products, as well as post-marketing surveys. The team recognised that that they did not give sufficient attention to the views and needs of a range of healthcare workers and did not review their educational strategy, but reproduced standard promotional material without consideration of the target audience. However, the study by Rao *et al.* 2002 was able to demonstrate a 17.4% reduction in the incidence of *C. difficile*-associated diarrhoea (CDAD) and an 11% reduction in the number of nosocomial cases of MRSA. As noted by Pittet (2000), behavioural theories and interventions have largely targeted the individual, but consideration should also be given to environmental issues, as well as the institutional climate.

Mah, Deshpand and Rothschild (2006) and others (Haley, Culver and White 1985; Jenner and Wilson 2000, King 2005) noted that changing health-care worker behaviour is a core function of infection-control programmes. However, Mah *et al.* (2006) suggests that the social change technologies of education and institutional policy are limited in their capacity to achieve sustained improvements in areas such as hand hygiene (Pittet *et al.* 2000) or barrier precautions (Larsen and Kretzer 1995). Mah *et al.* (2006) indicated that an educational approach offered the healthcare worker freedom to choose compliance, but also maximised the potential for increased morbidity, mortality, colonisation and loss of productivity arising from costs to patients, or the health system, through non-adherence. This may seem a harsh interpretation, but undoubtedly the position has credibility even though it can be difficult to quantify. This paper (Mah *et al.* 2006) observed that institutional policy can induce non-voluntary behaviour through threat of punishment or sanctions, but the threat of punishment cannot influence behaviour if a healthcare worker lacks the opportunity or ability to act in the correct manner. It also has the added risk of damaging cooperation between staff and management.

Mah *et al.* (2006) proposed a model of social marketing that addressed such problems of lack of time, inaccessible sinks, lack of knowledge or skin irritation, and suggested an approach that could make a change in behaviour seem easy, possible and attractive through promotion of the benefits to the individual and by providing opportunities to perform the activity. This would then benefit not only the employee but also the organisation and stakeholders, such as patients.

As Jenner *et al.* (2005) noted, messages around infection control have tended towards 'telling' rather than 'selling' and perhaps it is time that infection-control practitioners were more aware of human motivators such as 'self-interest' in the performance of certain practices. A study in Canada (Mah *et al.* 2005) noted that personal health was a stronger motivator of immunisation participation against influenza than the perceived benefits to patients.

Marketing perspectives suggest that benefits are considered more attractive if they are tangible, certain, direct and immediate (Mah, Deshpand and Rothschild 2006). Interventions such as fitting alcohol dispensers at the bedside to make hand decontamination easier could be supported by marketing strategies indicating that even busy healthcare workers would find hand rubs fast and effective at killing superbugs on their hands and this could be viewed as a gain to the worker, patients and clients.

CONCLUSION

When developing strategies to improve compliance with infection control activity, wider insights into human motivation and perception and use of marketing techniques must be employed to offer gains rather than losses to healthcare workers.

In the UK, social marketing has successfully been applied to the use of seat belts, motor cycle helmets, smoking in public places and the use of mobile phones when driving. It is an important technique when used in conjunction with education and policy to address behaviour change in the practice of infection prevention and control.

REFERENCES

BBC News. Superbug deaths triple in region. 2007. Available at: http://news.bbc.co.uk/1/hi/england/nottinghamshire/6386501.stm (accessed 25 Nov 2008).

Bloom B. *Taxonomy of Educational Objectives.* Boston: Allyn & Bacon; 1956.

Boyce J. It is time for action: improving hand hygiene in hospitals. *Ann Intern Med.* 1999; 130: 153–5.

British Medical Association (BMA). *Medicine in the 21st Century.* London: British Medical Association; 2005.

Chalmers C, Straub M. Standard principles for preventing and controlling infection. *Nurs Stand.* 2006; 20(23): 57–65.

Cole M. Using a motivational paradigm to improve handwashing compliance. *Nurse Educ Pract.* 2006; 6: 156–62.

Department of Health. *Hospital Infection Control: guidance in the control of infection in hospitals.* London: Public Health Laboratory Service; 1995.

Department of Health. *The NHS Plan: a plan for investment; a plan for reform.* London: Department of Health; 2000.

Department of Health. *Winning Ways: working together to reduce healthcare associated infection in England.* London: Department of Health; 2003.

Department of Health. *Infection Control Training for Over 1 million Staff.* Press Release. London: Department of Health; 4 Nov 2004.

Department of Health. *Action on Healthcare-Associated Infection in England.* London: Department of Health; 2005.

Department of Health. *Going Further Faster: implementing the saving lives delivery programme.* London: Department of Health; 2006.

Dewey J. *Experience and Education.* London: Macmillan; 1963.

DHSS. *Guidelines on Control of Hospital Infection.* London: DHSS; 1988.

Duckworth G. Controlling methicillin-resistant *Staphyloccoccus aureus. BMJ.* 2003; **327**: 1177–8.

Gallaher A, Holland L. Work-based learning challenges and opportunities. *Nurs Stand.* 2004; **19**: 39–42.

General Medical Council (GMC). *Setting Standards Codes of Conduct.* London: General Medical Council; 2006.

Haley RW, Culver DH, White JW. The efficacy of infection surveillance and control programs in preventing nosocomial infection in US hospitals. *Am J Epidemiol.* 1985; **21**: 183–205.

Health Professions Council (HPC). *Standards for Continuing Professional Development.* 2005. Available at: www.hpc-uk.org/registrants/cpd/ (accessed 25 Nov 2008).

Horton R. Linking the chain. *Nurs Times.* 1988; **84**(26): 44–6.

Huggonet S, Perneger T, Pittet D. Alcohol hand rub improves compliance with hand hygiene in intensive care units. *Arch Intern Med.* 2002; **162**: 1037–43.

Jenner EA, Jones F, Fletcher B, *et al.* Hand hygiene posters: selling the message. *J Hosp Infect.* 2005; **59**(2): 77–82.

Jenner EA, Wilson J. Educating the infection control team: past, present and future: a British perspective. *J Hosp Infect.* 2000; **46**: 96–105.

Karabey SA, Derbentli S, Nakipoglu Y, *et al.* Handwashing frequencies in an intensive care unit. *J Hosp Infect.* 2002; **50**: 36–41.

King D. Development of core competencies for infection prevention and control. *Nurs Stand.* 2005; **19**(41): 50–4.

Knappett CR. Infection control organisation in hospitals in England and Wales, 1979. *Health Trends.* 1981; **13**: 93–6.

Larsen E, Kretzer EK. Compliance with hand washing and barrier precautions. *J Hosp Infect.* 1995; **30**(Suppl.): 88–106.

Larsen EL, Early E, Cloonan P, *et al.* An organisational climate intervention associated with increased hand washing and decreased nosocomial infections. *Behav Med.* 2000; **26**: 14–22.

McCulloch J. Infection control principles for practice. *Nurs Stand.* 1998; **13**: 49–56.

MacDonald A, Dinah F, MacKenzie D, *et al.* Performance feedback of hand hygiene using alcohol hand gel as the skin decontaminant reduces the number of patients newly affected by MRSA and antibiotic costs. *J Hosp Infect.* 2004; **56**(1): 56–63.

McGuckin M. Evaluation of patient empowering hand hygiene programme. *J Hosp Infect.* 2001; **48**(3): 222–7.

McGuckin M, Waterman R, Porten L, *et al.* Patient education model for increasing hand hygiene compliance. *Am J Infect Control.* 1999; **27**(4): 309–14.

McIntosh K. Hospitals at risk of MRSA liability. *Nurs Times.* 2005; **101**(31): 4.

Mah MW, Deshpande S, Rothschild ML. Social marketing: a behaviour change technology for infection control. *Am J Infect Control.* 2006; **34**(7): 452–7.

Mah MW, Hagen NA, Pauling-Shepherd K, *et al.* Understanding influenza vaccination attitudes at a Canadian cancer centre. *Am J Infect Control.* 2005; **33**(4): 243–50.

Naikoba S, Hayward A. The effectiveness of interventions aimed at increasing hand washing in healthcare workers. *J Hosp Infect.* 2001; **29**(3): 173–80.

National Audit Office. *Management and Control of Hospital-Acquired Infection in Acute Trusts in England.* 17 Feb HC230. London: National Audit Office; 2000.

National Audit Office. *Improving Patient Care by Reducing Risks of Hospital-Acquired Infection.* Progress Report 14 July HC876. London: National Audit Office; 2004.

Nursing and Midwifery Council. *Standards of Proficiency for Pre-Registration Nursing Education.* 2004. Available at: www.nmc-uk.org (accessed 25 Nov 2008).

Nursing and Midwifery Council. *Code of Professional Conduct Performance and Ethics.* 2008. Available at: www.nmc-uk.org (accessed 25 Nov 2008).

Nursing and Midwifery Council. *The PREP Handbook Standards.* 2006. Available at: www.nmc-uk.org (accessed 25 Nov 2008).

Osbourne S. Influences on compliance with standard precautions among operating room nurses. *Am J Infect Control.* 2003; **31**(7): 415–23.

Pellowe CM, Pratt RJ, Loveday HP, *et al.* The EPIC project updating the evidence based guidelines for preventing healthcare associated infections in NHS hospitals in England. *Br J Infect Control.* 2004; **5**(6): 10–15.

Perry C. The infection control nurse past, present and future. *Br J Infect Control.* 2005; **16**(5): 18–21.

Pittet D. Improving compliance with hand hygiene. *Infect Cont Hosp Ep.* 2000; **21**: 381–6.

Pittet D. Infection control and quality healthcare in the new millennium. *Am J Infect Control.* 2005; **33**(5): 258–67.

Pittet D, Hugonnet S, Harbarth S, *et al.* Effectiveness of a hospital-wide programme to improve compliance with hand hygiene. *Lancet.* 2000; **356**(9238): 1307–12.

Randle J, Clarke E, Storr J. Hand hygiene compliance in healthcare workers. *J Hosp Infect.* 2006; **64**(3): 205–9.

Rao G, Jeanes A, Osman M, *et al.* Marketing hand hygiene in hospitals. *J Hosp Infect.* 2002; **50**(1): 42–7.

Senge P, Kleiner A, Roberts C, *et al. The Dance of Change: the challenges of maintaining momentum in learning organisations.* London: Nicholas Brealey Publishing; 1999.

Sheng WH, Wang JT, Lo DCT, *et al.* Comparative impact of hospital-acquired infection on medical costs, length of stay and outcome between community hospital and medical centres. *J Hosp Infect.* 2005; **59**: 205–14.

Storr J, Clayton-Kent S. Hand hygiene. *Nurs Stand.* 2004; **18**: 45–52 and 54.

Sud H, Gorman J. A nurse-led initiative to reduce levels of healthcare-associated infection in hospital. *Nurs Times.* 2007; **103**(14): 30–1.

Triggle N. MRSA superbug claims may surge. *BBC News.* 2006. Available at: http://news.bbc.co.uk/1/hi/health/6148546.stm (accessed 25 Nov 2008).

United Kingdom Health Department, Expert Advisory Group on AIDS and Expert Advisory Group on Hepatitis. *Guidance for Clinical Healthcare Workers Protection Against Infection with Blood-Borne Viruses.* London: Department of Health; 1998.

Walsh K. Blended learning. *BMJ.* 2005; **330**: 829.

Williams T. Patient empowerment and ethical decision making: the patient partner and the right to act. *Dimens Crit Care Nurs.* 2002; **21**(3): 100–5.

Wilson L, Greaves N. Why we need an NHS culture change to implement ICT change successfully and to give people modernised healthcare services. *Br J Healthcare Comput Info Manage.* 2002; **19**(8): 29–30 and 33.

CHAPTER 12

Challenging the status quo

My intention within this chapter is to reflect upon two questions:

1 Why is it important to challenge the status quo?
2 Why do health and social care professionals fail to do this as much as they should?

What do you think the two questions above have to do with reducing healthcare-acquired infection rates?

I present a number of related examples which have implications for safe infection control practice where the status quo should be challenged, but is not. Within these examples I shall draw upon my own experiences and those of others.

The two questions above are of considerable significance, based upon current levels of healthcare-acquired infection rates (Graves *et al.* 2007), the need to protect patients and clients from the harm infections can cause (Storr, Topley and Privett 2005) and the fact that as health and social care professionals we are a primary cause of cross infection (Stone *et al.* 2004) through, for example, poor adherence to hand hygiene. If health and social care professionals fail to challenge the status quo, unsafe practice will continue unabated – the consequences of which will be:

➤ harm occurring to patients, clients, their relatives and the health and social care professionals themselves;

➤ cross-infection rates continuing to rise;

➤ health and social care professionals continuing to breach the human rights of patients, clients and colleagues;

➤ breaches of health and safety continuing to occur.

➤ resources continuing to be stretched in the form of delays in discharging patients or clients creating extra financial and staffing demands;

➤ increased need for additional financial resources;

➤ lack of physical resources because finances are re-directed elsewhere;

➤ continued staff shortages as a result of finances being re-directed elsewhere.

As health and social care professionals, a fundamental aspect of our role is to challenge the status quo. That is, to ask at least two questions within a reflective framework (*see* Reflection exercise 12.2), 'Why?' and 'Who says so?' All too often health and social care professionals apply dissonance-based excuses (*see* Explanation box 12,1) to justify aspects of practice that are clearly unsafe, outdated and outmoded. For example, ritualistic beliefs which centre around, 'We have always done it that way so why change?' Such attitudes continue to exist within a variety of infection-control related situations.

REFLECTION EXERCISE 12.2

A reflective framework:

In reality, reflection is a complex cognitive process, but it can be summarised as being where an individual thinks about a past experience and applies their conclusions to facilitate their future development and practice. However, in order to undertake this process, which can be challenging, it is often useful to have a framework to follow.

Key word:	Explanatory statements:
Who?	Who was involved? What influence might they have had?
What?	What happened?
When?	When did the situation occur? Could this have influenced the outcome?
Where?	What was the environment? Could this have had an influence?
How?	How did you feel about what happened? What was positive and what could have been improved?

Why?   Why do you feel things went the way they did? What was your involvement and how might your presence have influenced things?

(Extracts from Elliott in Jasper 2006)

The answers to these questions are your personal thoughts and feelings about a given situation. However, how do you know that what you thought happened was correct?

In answer to this, you may say 'I do!' But how valid and reliable are your feelings and opinions?

Could there have been other interpretations of the event or situation you are reflecting upon?

EXPLANATION BOX 12.1 COGNITIVE DISSONANCE (FESTINGER 1962)

The concept of cognitive dissonance was originally identified by Festinger (1962), where he proposed that, at a psychological level, the individual will strive to make consistent two or more things that would not naturally be so. In simple terms, dissonance effects are when an individual generates excuses to justify their previous behaviour or behaviour they wish or intend to carry out. Hand hygiene is a good example, where the individual understands its importance in reducing cross infection, yet fails to adequately follow the hand hygiene process. Thus the individual experiences conflict between knowing what they should do and what they actually do or want to do.

Such conflict would be manifested as stress in the individual and in an attempt to reduce such stress the individual will generate an excuse or reason for failing to follow the hand hygiene process. Such an excuse may be blamed on time, work load or an irrational belief that meeting other's needs must take priority over undertaking standard precautions. In reality the meeting of others needs must include undertaking standard precautions.

WHY CHALLENGE THE STATUS QUO?

The following examples are aspects of practice where infection control is a factor, but where the status quo is rarely, if ever, challenged.

The chain of infection

The chain of infection (*see* List 12.1) is a biomedically-based model (*see* List 12.2) used extensively by health and social care professionals.

LIST 12.1 COMPONENTS OF THE CHAIN OF INFECTION

The chain of infection is made up of various components:

1 Infectious agent: health and social care professionals.
2 Reservoirs – environmental: physical objects, enclosed spaces where close proximity exists between people.
3 Portals of entry to the person: wounds, inhalation, physical contact, ingestion.
4 Portals of exit from the person: coughing, sneezing, elimination, wounds.
5 Susceptible host: recipients of healthcare and other members of the general population who enter and exit healthcare establishments.
6 Mode of transmission: failure to undertake preventative measures and acts of omission; disregard of standard precautions.

In its current format, the chain of infection only reflects physical factors related to the nature of cross infection. However, as has been identified in Chapter 4,

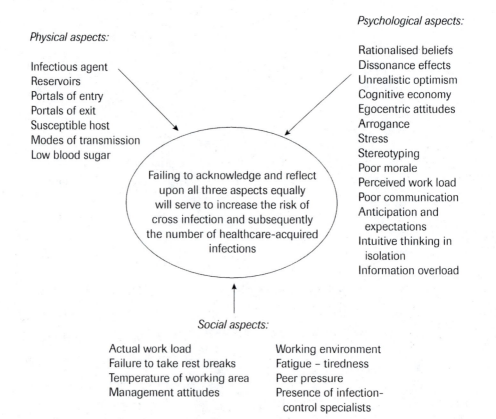

Physical aspects:

Infectious agent
Reservoirs
Portals of entry
Portals of exit
Susceptible host
Modes of transmission
Low blood sugar

Psychological aspects:

Rationalised beliefs
Dissonance effects
Unrealistic optimism
Cognitive economy
Egocentric attitudes
Arrogance
Stress
Stereotyping
Poor morale
Perceived work load
Poor communication
Anticipation and
  expectations
Intuitive thinking in
  isolation
Information overload

Failing to acknowledge and reflect upon all three aspects equally will serve to increase the risk of cross infection and subsequently the number of healthcare-acquired infections

Social aspects:

Actual work load
Failure to take rest breaks
Temperature of working area
Management attitudes

Working environment
Fatigue – tiredness
Peer pressure
Presence of infection-
  control specialists

FIGURE 12.1 A unified approach to the causal nature of cross infection.

there is no empirical evidence to support the chain of infection's successful application. In addition, information relating to the chain of infection's origins is somewhat spurious. Clearly, in its current form, this model is questionable regarding the contribution it makes towards reducing rising cross-infection rates. Furthermore it cannot be described as holistic in its approach to instilling an understanding that there are physical, psychological and social reasons why cross infection occurs (Figure 12.1). Yet health and social care professionals and healthcare providers continue to adopt this model, which is clearly outdated and outmoded and, as such, is unreliable.

REFLECTION EXERCISE 12.3

Can you think of a situation where the chain of infection has been successful in reducing levels of cross infection or non-adherence to standard precautions?

In what ways do you feel the chain of infection could be made more holistic and less biomedically orientated?

In thinking about this you may want to take another look at Chapter 4.

Lack of contact with patients

Where many health and social professionals are concerned, their generalised lack of contact with patients or clients has implications for the degree to which standard precautions are adhered to. As Teale (2007) indicates, many professionals only instigate direct contact with patients or clients when it is necessary to carry out a specific task. Therefore, with direct contact being minimal and task-orientated, health and social care professionals will have a greater propensity to believe that consistent adoption of standard precautions is not necessary. However, such a belief is consistent with a biomedical approach (*see* List 12.2) and an external locus of control (*see* Explanation box 12.2). Furthermore, such a belief can be seen as a consequence of cognitively economic thinking (Explanation box 12.3).

EXPLANATION BOX 12.2 HEALTH LOCUS OF CONTROL (WALLSTON AND WALLSTON 1982; ADAMS AND BROMLEY 1998)

Locus of control consists of two dimensions:

1 Internal: This is the partnership between the patient or client and the healthcare worker, whether it be professional, administrative, managerial or ancillary. Such partnerships reflect the provision of information, non-judgemental attitudes and the right to ask questions without fear of

ridicule and retribution. Such an approach is reflective of a biopsychosocial perspective.

Example: With regard to standard precautions, patients and clients have the right to have their questions answered in order for them to make informed choices as to whether they wish to comply with the advice given by healthcare workers.

2 External: This is where the patient or client is expected to be unquestioning, compliant and submissive to the demands of healthcare workers. Such an approach is reflective of a biomedical perspective.

Example: With regard to standard precautions, patients and clients are denied the opportunity to ensure that these are appropriately applied within the context of their healthcare experience.

EXPLANATION BOX 12.3 COGNITIVE ECONOMY
(ROTH AND FRISBY 1992)

Cognitive economy is where an individual has become context-specific or tunnel-visioned in their perception of what is occurring around them and will fail to take into account the wider implications of their behaviour. For example, instead of being patient-centred, the individual will become task-orientated towards achieving a set of goals that will meet their own needs at the expense of everything else and the needs of others.

Example: In the case of standard precautions, the individual will be context-specific towards achieving their allocated work load and as a result of this may:
- fail to change their gloves between interventions;
- fail to undertake or to fully follow the hand hygiene process;
- fail to ensure that they have removed all the equipment they used following completion of a procedure.

LIST 12.2 RELATING THE BIOMEDICAL
MODEL TO INFECTION CONTROL

This model (Elliott and BVS Training 2005) assumes that:
1 The concepts of health and illness are seen to exist separately.
Infection control example: Healthcare-acquired infection and the interventions

made by health and social care professionals are seen as existing in isolation, but they are not perceived as impacting upon each other.

2 Disease or infection is external to the body and is not the result of an individual's behaviour.

Infection control example: The behaviour of health and social care professionals has no impact upon the risk of cross infection.

3 Individuals should have no control over or involvement with what happens to them regarding their health and wellbeing.

Infection control example: Patients and clients have no right to question or challenge health and social care professionals even though they may have contracted a healthcare-acquired infection through the health or social care professional's negligence as a result of their poor or inadequate adoption of standard precautions.

4 Individuals have no responsibility to ensure the maintenance of their own or others' health and wellbeing.

Infection control example: Despite failing to adopt standard precautions, health and social care professionals are not responsible for the consequences of such a failure.

5 Although it is acknowledged they exist, the mind and body are perceived as being separate with neither having consequences for the other.

Infection control example: A health and social care professional who is experiencing stress will demonstrate a greater propensity towards becoming cognitively economic (*see* Explanation box 12.3) and unrealistically optimistic (*see* Explanation box 12.4) in their perception of the importance of standard precautions. Despite this, there will be no impact upon their behaviour; therefore, a failure to carry out standard precautions according to a bio-medical perspective is not a consequence of the way a health or social care professional thinks but simply a physical action.

6 Psychosocial factors have no part to play and healthcare intervention should centre around the physical aspects in isolation.

Infection control example: Healthcare-acquired infection has nothing to do with how health and social care professionals think or the social context within which they are practising. Cross infection is simply a consequence of physical factors, such as the cleanliness of equipment, the environment or staff uniforms/work clothing.

7 Health and social care professionals are knowledgeable experts who always know best.

Infection control example: Attitudes such as, 'I am safe', 'I am competent', 'I know what I am doing' or 'I am an expert' are all indicative of dissonance-based thinking (*see* Explanation box 12.1) and a cognitively economic perspective (*see* Explanation box 12.3) towards their ability to carry out consistent safe infection control practice. However, terms such as 'safe', 'competent' and 'expert' are all spurious in nature and are reflective of an egocentric and conceited self-perception, which serves to precipitate unsafe infection-control behaviour.

8   Patients and clients cease to have their own identity. Rather they become stereotyped or labelled by health and social care professionals.
Infection control example: Patients and clients who contract a healthcare-acquired infection may be seen as the health problem they present within isolation, as opposed to a person in their own right. For example, a patient with MRSA loses the right to be seen as a person and becomes an entity. This entity principle has particular relevance when a patient or client having contracted a healthcare-acquired infection is placed in a side room, becomes perceived as dirty and is then forgotten – out of sight and out of mind!

9   It is acceptable to ridicule a patient or client when they fail to conform to the assumptions, expectations or requirements of health and social care professionals.
Infection control example: Patients and clients who experience a healthcare-acquired infection become stigmatised by health and social care professionals who may originally have been responsible for them contracting an infection in the first place. As a result of such they are perceived as failing to conform with the expectations of those health and social care professionals.

NB: The above should not be seen as being mutually exclusive, but rather as providing a perspective.

For example, any health or social care professional who believes that the risks of cross infection are governed by the level of direct contact with patients or clients is clearly cognitively economic (*see* Explanation box 12.3) in their perspective. In such a situation a consequence of being cognitively economic would enhance dissonance effects (*see* Explanation box 12.1) and health and social care professionals would become unrealistically optimistic (*see* Explanation box 12.4) regarding the nature of cross infection and routes of transmission.

EXPLANATION BOX 12.4 UNREALISTIC OPTIMISM (OGDEN 2007)

Unrealistic optimism is where a health or social care professional becomes unrealistically optimistic regarding the risky situation they place themselves and others in as a result of behaviour that constitutes unsafe infection control practice in the form of failing to undertake standard precautions or through failing to follow the hand hygiene process.

Unrealistic optimism can be facilitated through lack of personal experience. For example, a health or social care professional who has no prior experience of a patient's or client's health being directly influenced by their failure to adopt appropriate standard precautions will likely believe two things (Elliott 2003):

1   There is no risk, or the risk of cross infecting others is so insignificant that it simply does not matter.
2   Even if there is a risk it will not happen to them. That is, even if the individual involved in healthcare does cross infect others they will rationalise that is was not their fault (*see* Explanation box 12.1) or they will not be found out and held responsible and therefore, who cares?

A lack of patient or client contact on the part of health and social care professionals can be seen as a causal factor for non-adherence to standard precautions resulting from attitudes such as:

1   If I do not go near the patients or clients then I am not spreading infection.
2   By only going to the patient or client when they need something, I am helping to reduce the risk of cross infection.
3   I have not got the time to keep checking on the patients or clients as I have too much administration to do. Anyway handling paper work, pens and computer keyboards does not contribute to cross infection. Cross infection only occurs when I go near patients or clients.
4   Of course I am person-centred in the care I give. When something needs doing I get it done as quickly as possible and therefore I am reducing the risk of cross infection.
5   Speed is the important thing; get in and out as quickly as possible so the infection does not have a chance to spread.
6   My role only requires me to talk to patients or clients and not to touch them; therefore, if I do not touch the patient or client I cannot be responsible for cross infection.

How much contact with your patients and clients do you have?

Do you only make contact with them as is indicated by Teale (2007), when there is a specific task to carry out?

Are you person-centred or task-orientated in the way you interact with patients and clients?

Wearing coats over work clothing

Some health and social care workers believe that wearing a coat over their work clothing will reduce the risk of cross infection. Within some healthcare settings this dissonance-based behaviour (*see* Explanation box 12.1) is seen to occur with amazing regularity. An example is when theatre staff wear a white coat when leaving the operating-department setting to visit the hospital shop.

The following two examples relate to my own experiences where coats and staff behaviour clearly constituted infection control violations.

While on a recent visit to a southeast England regional general hospital, I observed an individual walking down a corridor in their theatre attire and a white coat, which was wide open. Clearly this coat was having no impact upon the potential for preventing cross infection. However, what was that even more concerning and clearly reflective of dissonance-based (*see* Explanation box 12.1) and cognitively economic thinking (*see* Explanation box 12.3) was that when I casually asked this individual why they were wearing a white coat their response was 'It protects me from carrying infection because I am only away from theatres for a short while.' This might also reflect attitudes held by operating department staff who were found to be taking cigarette breaks outside the operating room – in their theatre attire – between surgical cases (O'Dowd 2006).

The second example relates to my being in a queue to be served behind an individual in operating theatre attire who was wearing an open white coat within a regional hospital on the south coast of England. As we progressed to the till, this individual found themselves standing next to a basket of fruit. At this point they started to pick up the apples and sniff each one before replacing it in the basket.

Both of these experiences reflect shocking examples of behaviour where the public could have been placed at risk. Furthermore, within the context of health and safety, they could well have constituted a failure to maintain the health and welfare of others. The behaviour of these two individuals also demonstrates the impact psychological factors can play in increasing the potential for cross infection to occur.

A further example where such dissonance-based ritualistic beliefs seem inherent is where health and social care professionals choose to travel home in their work clothes, but believe that by covering their work clothes with a coat it will serve to reduce or prevent cross infection. On many occasions' health and social care professionals wear coats that are open, over work clothing whilst shopping and handling unprotected foods in food retail outlets. Such behaviour is clearly in contravention to that set out in professional codes of conduct and the guidelines of some professional bodies. For example, the Royal College of Nursing of the United Kingdom (2007) clearly identifies that staff should change out of their uniforms at the end of their working period. What is also worrying is that staff employed by food retailers appear oblivious to the dangers of such behaviour. Health and social care professionals who are wearing their work clothing should be barred access to retailers who sell foods.

REFLECTION EXERCISE 12.5

Have you ever worn your work clothing to go shopping at the end of your working period?

If you have, how much of a cross-infection risk do you think you were creating by wearing clothing that may be contaminated?

Regular imposition of prescriptive rules

The regular imposition of prescriptive rules is also a practice that has become ritualised within health and social care almost to the point of 'if in doubt write a policy or procedure that everyone must adhere to'. However, the logic of such an approach, where there is a belief among many in health and social care that people will simply adhere to a rule is dissonance-based (*see* Explanation box 12.1), cognitively economic (*see* Explanation box 12.3) and unrealistically optimistic (*see* Explanation box 12.4) in the extreme. It has been indicated (Lawton and Parker 1999, 2002; Reason, Parker and Lawton 1998) that such prescriptive rules are not the answer where promoting safe practice is concerned. For example, most healthcare providers have an infection-control policy in place and readily available to their employees. Yet where the provision of such a policy is measured against non-adherence to standard precautions, clearly the impact of the policy is at best minimal because staff have never read the policy or they read it so long ago that they can not remember its content. Despite this, health and social care providers continue to place heavy reliance on such rules as a means of controlling unsafe behaviour (Elliott 2003; Grilli and Lomas 1994).

Do you always comply with your employer's policies and procedures?

If not, why not?

Can you think of reasons why you do not adhere to rules that exist for your protection and if you are caught not adhering to them you should be subject to disciplinary action?

When colleagues fail to adhere to standard precautions

Where a health or social care professional observes a colleague failing to adhere to standard precautions (*see* List 12.3) it is likely they will do a variety of things:

➤ selectively ignore the behaviour;

➤ follow what their colleague does and particularly so if that person is someone they believe to be more knowledgeable or powerful than they are;

➤ say nothing to the colleague, but be critical of them behind their back or generate a dissonance-based excuse to justify their colleague's behaviour.

LIST 12.3 STANDARD PRECAUTIONS

There are a number of standard precautions involved in infection control:

1 **Recognising the need** to adopt standard precautions is the most important aspect. Failing to recognise the need is governed by the way an individual thinks, which will, in turn, impact upon their perception of the relevance and importance of such precautions. If an individual perceives standard precautions as being irrelevant, unimportant or of a lesser priority, then the potential for non-adherence is significantly increased.

2 **Hand hygiene** is vital in facilitating the prevention and reduction of healthcare-acquired infections. Hand hygiene must be carried out frequently by individuals who are constantly reflecting upon the principle of what they have just done and what they are about to do now. If the *just done* constitutes a risk to themselves or others then appropriate hand hygiene must be undertaken prior to proceeding to the *do now*. Also, consideration must be given to the full hand hygiene process.

3 **Hand cleansing rubs/gels** are an effective method of hand decontamination in the short term. However, they should never be perceived as an absolute substitute for the adoption of formal hand hygiene using the hand hygiene process.

4 **Disposable aprons** can provide some protection for the wearer. However, they should never be perceived as an absolute barrier and must be changed frequently. As a general rule the *just done, do now* approach should be adopted at all times.

5 **Disposable gloves** must always be worn when handling body fluids or any contaminated substance/materials. As a general rule, if in doubt wear gloves. Management and/or colleagues should not presume to ridicule or restrict an individual's decision to wear gloves.

6 **Skin trauma** must be dealt with in accordance with the employer's policies and procedures, and in accordance with health and safety laws. All trauma to the skin, irrespective of how minor, must be cleaned, dried, covered and reported. It is a legal requirement that an accident/incident form is completed and individuals should report to either the Occupational Health Department or to Accident and Emergency.

7 **The eyes** should be protected where there is either a potential or actual risk of flying debris or splashes of body fluids/harmful substances. Individuals must determine for themselves when the wearing of appropriate eye protection is necessary. Management should not presume to restrict such determinations or they may be in contravention of an individual's human rights under Articles 1 and 10 (Wilkinson and Caulfield 2001).

8 **Sharps** are dangerous and will cause harm. A sharp may be defined as anything that can either penetrate or cause trauma to the skin. An injury from a sharp may have consequences for the remainder of an individual's life. Always handle sharps with caution for your own safety and that of those around you. The rule is that if you have been using sharps then you are responsible to clear up what you have used and dispose of the sharps correctly. If you do not do this you are acting in an unprofessional and unethical manner.

9 **Spillages** of any kind can be hazardous to the health and wellbeing of you and others. The rule is, if you cause the spillage then you clean it up or ensure it is dealt with in the correct way. Your employer's policies and procedures for dealing with spillages must be adhered to at all times.

10 **Waste materials** can be divided into three categories: household, clinical and contaminated/hazardous. However, all categories of waste should be handled with caution as each one is capable of increasing the risk of cross infection and causing harm to yourself and others. Your employer's policies and procedures for the disposal of waste must be adhered to at all times.

11 **Linen**, like waste materials, must be handled with care due to the increased potential for cross infection. When handling soiled or contaminated linen appropriate protective clothing should be worn. With regard to the handling

of clean linen, the *just done, do now* approach should be adopted. Your employer's policies and procedures for the handling of linen must be adhered to at all times.

12 **Food handling** is an activity that we all do either at a personal level for our own consumption or at a social level for consumption by others. The mishandling of food is a prime source of cross infection and the use of appropriate protective clothing and meticulous hand hygiene is essential using the *just done, do now* approach.

13 **Environmental contamination**, although not always visible to the human eye, is always present. Therefore regular and rigorous cleaning of healthcare environments is essential to reduce the risk of cross infection. Although many people involved in the provision of healthcare perceive such environmental cleaning as being the role of designated cleaners, such a role is arguably the responsibility of everyone. The rule is that if you cause the contamination, you clean it up or ensure it is cleaned up in an appropriate manner. It is both unethical and unprofessional to simply leave contamination with the expectation that it is someone else's responsibility to clean it up.

14 **Personal hygiene** of those involved in the provision of healthcare and recipients of healthcare is an essential measure where the reduction of cross infection is concerned.

Stereotyping and labelling patients, clients and colleagues

Unfortunately, stereotyping and labelling patients, clients and colleagues is something that is entrenched in the behaviour of health and social care professionals. This is because stereotyping and labelling are ways of categorising our feelings and attitudes about people. However, the ways in which we categorise others can be very negative and have destructive effects upon the individuals at which it is directed. For example, intelligence is a concept that we use to determine an individual's abilities, according to what each of us believes they should be capable of doing. We make these judgements based upon our observations of others' behaviour and then categorise their degree of intelligence accordingly. For example, if in the past you have been conversing with a colleague or patient/client who repeatedly fails to grasp what you were attempting to communicate to them, what did you subsequently think about them and what did you say about them behind their back? The chances are your thoughts and statements about them may have been less than complimentary. Yet if you were to find yourself in a similar situation, would you consider yourself to be of low intelligence or stupid just because you could not understand or grasp what was being communicated to you? Almost certainly not. As such, those health and social care professionals who apply such labels are, in effect, being hypocritical.

The way we allocate intelligence tends to happen as a generalisation. That is, the individual is either intelligent or not; the individual is either stupid or not; or the individual is either competent or not. However, such a generalisation will impact upon the way you behave towards a given individual. If you perceive them to be unintelligent, stupid or incompetent, then your communication towards them will change and you will be more likely to adopt a condescending approach. An example of this is with the elderly, where just because an individual is mature in years and may be a little deaf we feel the need to talk down to them and treat them in the same way we would a child or an individual in a wheel chair who is experiencing a health problem and who has a carer with them. Who more often than not is the one the health or social care professional communicates with? Answer: the carer – which is both unprofessional and unethical.

REFLECTION EXERCISE 12.7

With regards to the two examples above, have you ever behaved in such a way to another individual?

If your response is yes, how ethical and professional was your behaviour?

If your response is no, what are your feelings about the ethics and professionalism of those who do behave in such ways?

Within the context of infection control, non-adherence to standard precautions could occur as a result of a health or social care professional adopting stereotypical attitudes like 'They're old and deaf and won't notice if I don't wash my hands. Anyway what does it matter? They will be gone soon.' At this point you may be horrified by such a statement but I challenge you to contact me and deny that such attitudes do not exist in healthcare.

However, if a broader approach to the nature of intelligence is adopted, it may serve to reduce such generalisations, which, in turn, may reduce non-adherence to standard precautions through each of us becoming more self-aware. This type of broader approach can be seen in the works of Gardner *et al.* (cited in Atkinson *et al.* 2000). Instead of seeing intelligence as a thing that people have or do not, Gardner *et al.* proposes seven types of intelligence (List 12.4).

LIST 12.4 MULTIPLE INTELLIGENCE

The information below should be seen as not being mutually exclusive, but as examples formulated from that presented within Gardner *et al.* cited in Atkinson *et al.* (2000).

1 Linguistic intelligence – the ability to understand:
   ● sounds;
   ● the rules by which words are formed and put together;
   ● the interrelationship between words, phrases and sentences.
2 Musical intelligence – the ability to:
   ● use of the imagination and create new ideas or things;
   ● converse, correspond, impart and share;
   ● infer meaning from sounds.
3 Logic/mathematical intelligence – the ability to:
   ● understand concepts and relationship between concepts.
4 Spatial intelligence – the ability to:
   ● understand events in time and space.
5 Bodily/kinesthetic intelligence – the ability to:
   ● use our bodies to problem solve, involving motor actions and the manipulation of objects.
6 Intrapersonal intelligence – the ability to:
   ● distinguish between our emotions, our intentions, our desires and our moral conscience.
7 Interpersonal intelligence – the ability to:
   ● recognise and accept others' attitudes, values and beliefs – even if they are different from your own.

The point here is that we are all intelligent, but in different ways. However, where Gardner offers seven types of intelligence, in reality there could be an infinite number of intelligences; for example, the ability to drive a car, play a musical instrument or the ability to understand another person speaking with an accent or in a different language. Therefore, as health and social care professionals, if we adopt such an approach it can serve to reduce negative attitudes like the one above with regards to the adoption of standard precautions. In essence, the way we think, which is a reflection of our attitudes, can affect our adoption of standard precautions in either a positive or negative way.

A second way in which health and social care professionals stereotype and label is through terminology in the form of jargon and titles as measures to determine roles. We use terminology as a method for identifying categories of people; for example, patient, client, service user, surgical, medical, a location or condition. Such terminology can impact upon the attitudes we hold and our behaviour towards others.

In some cases, the terminology we use can have very negative connotations. For example, if we consider the term 'patient' I wonder how many of you reading this are aware that it derives from a Latin verb that means 'to suffer or bear' (Neuberger 1999). It would seem to me that this puts a rather different perspective upon the way health and social care professionals use and apply the term 'patient'. If we consider this in the light of current rates of healthcare-acquired infection and mortality rates as a result of such infections, *to suffer* would seem to be quite representative of what we actually do to many of our patients, clients and colleagues through cross infecting them and of course they then have to *bear* the consequences of our actions or omissions. Furthermore, the current level of non-adherence to standard precautions within health and social care can only be interpreted as a conscious disregard for suffering created through our non-adherence.

REFLECTION EXERCISE 12.8

Think about situations where you have stereotyped or labelled others that affected the way you thought and felt about them. In addition, think about whether your thoughts and feelings about someone else affected your behaviour towards them, or in the case of a patient or client, affected the quality of care you gave them.

THE NEED TO CHALLENGE THE STATUS QUO

For each of the examples above, there is a need to challenge the status quo: the way we think, the attitudes we hold and our behaviour – all of which can have an impact upon the health and wellbeing of others and can serve to promote our non-adherence to the adoption of standard precautions. This is because if the way we think and our attitudes towards an individual are negative then it is likely that our behaviour towards that individual will also be negative. Furthermore, if we do not challenge the attitudes and unsafe behaviours of our colleagues then the individual may never be aware that what they are doing is unsafe.

Having read the above examples, how does it make you feel?

Are you guilty of such behaviour?

If your answer is yes, how are you feeling right now?

If your answer is no, can you think of any ritualised infection control-related behaviour that you have observed that would be consistent with the premise 'It has always been done that way so why change?'

I have shown clear examples of where the status quo needs to be challenged. Yet how often and to what extent do health and social care professionals actively and openly offer challenges to such behaviour? I would argue that the answer is rarely – if ever. None of the behaviours set out within the examples above are consistent with protecting patients, clients and the general population from harm or the philosophy of *do no harm*. However, by failing to challenge the status quo where such behaviour is concerned, we are, albeit indirectly, doing harm, which may well contravene the principles that under-pin international health law (Taylor 2002) regarding:

➤ the transmission of communicable diseases;

➤ an individual's human rights (Wilkinson and Caulfield 2001);

➤ a health or social care professional's particular code of professional conduct.

With regard to health and safety at work, each of us is required to make every effort to maintain the health, safety and welfare of those within our workplace (Taylor 2002). Failing to do this can lead to legal action against not only the individual health or social care professional, but also their employer (*see* Chapter 3). In principle, an individual who fails to challenge the status quo is just as guilty of causing harm as the individual who, for example, fails to adopt appropriate hand hygiene.

Failing to change out of your work clothing prior to leaving your place of work could be seen as breaching the human rights of others under the Human Rights Act (1998), specifically Article 2 (The Right to Life) because you could through cross infection be denying them their life, Article 3 (Prohibition of Torture) through causing them physical, psychological or social pain, anxiety and distress and Article 5 (The Right to Liberty and Security) through causing them to have to remain in your care for longer than was necessary (Wilkinson and Caulfield 2001).

Where each health and social care professional's particular code of conduct and The Health Act (Department of Health 2006) are concerned, they both identify the need to protect patients, clients and those within the wider society.

As professionals, we should not only be challenging our own infection control-related behaviour, but also those of our colleagues at the point at which they occur. To wait until later to offer a challenge can have dangerous consequences for the safety of all. However, many health and social care workers believe themselves to be professional in what they do and to fit within what is socially perceived to constitute being a professional. Yet, in reflecting upon the generalised failure of many health and social care professionals to openly challenge the behaviour and attitudes of others when measured against definitions of the words 'professional' and 'unprofessional', it is evident that in failing to challenge the status quo we are behaving unprofessionally (*see* List 12.5).

LIST 12.5 COMPARISONS BETWEEN THE WORDS 'PROFESSIONAL' AND 'UNPROFESSIONAL' (WHERE 'PROFESSIONAL' EQUATES WITH CHALLENGING THE STATUS QUO)

Professional:	Unprofessional:
Skilled	Unethical
Proficient	Unprincipled
Knowledgeable	Immoral
Competent	Incompetent
Focused	Disreputable
Dedicated	Second-rate
Qualified	Inadequate
Intelligent	Dangerous
Trustworthy	Untrustworthy

WHY DO WE FAIL TO CHALLENGE THE STATUS QUO?

It is interesting that most health and social care workers know and understand the importance of challenging the status quo. Yet when confronted with situations that require such a challenge, individuals shy away from doing so. Therefore, I would like to offer some possible reasons and explanations for this apparent anomaly: where those in health and social care know what they should do, but in reality fail to do it (*see* List 12.6).

LIST 12.6 REASONS FOR FAILING TO CHALLENGE THE STATUS QUO

There are a variety of reasons for not challenging the status quo:
1 Fear of retribution.
2 Fear of being ostracised from a peer group.
3 Indifference and choosing to ignore what they observe.
4 'Not my responsibility.'
5 Low morale.
6 Low self esteem.
7 Low blood sugar through failing to take adequate nourishment and fluids during the working period.
8 Simply do not care.
9 Failing to regularly update knowledge base and thus not being aware when the status quo needs to be challenged.
10 Do not have the time.
11 Too busy meeting patients/clients needs.
12 Do not want to cause a fuss or upset anyone.
13 Lack of management support.

I would suggest one of the primary reasons individuals do not challenge the status quo is out of fear of retribution – either from the individual being challenged or from an employer. If you were to observe someone you recognised as holding authority over you or as being more senior to you failing to adopt appropriate standard precautions would you challenge their non-adherence? Even if you did, would you feel stressed and anxious about doing so? I suggest that in making your decision to challenge or not you would, in part, be influenced by your past experience of offering challenges. If the individual you challenged reacted in a positive fashion then it is likely that you would feel more confident about challenging in the future. For example, the challenged individual might respond by saying 'You're absolutely right and I stand corrected'.

From my own personal experience, many years ago whilst serving in the Royal Air Force and working in general practice, I became involved in a professional discussion with the Senior Medical Officer (who was considerably higher in rank than I). As a part of that discussion I remember saying to this senior officer: 'What is it that makes doctors feel they have the right to always assume they should be the leader of a team?' Having made this comment (and if I am honest then wishing the ground would open up and swallow me!), I received a reply to the effect of 'No one. You just let us! Perhaps you should not do so.' Now at this point – and having made the comment, half expecting to be charged, marched to the guardroom under escort and the key to the cell thrown away – I felt much relief at their response and that it was so positive. What I also felt, and which was subsequently confirmed by the medical officer, was that they recognised that my comment was made within the context of 'seeking to develop'. There is no doubt that positive responses from those we challenge will serve to facilitate our future development and how willing we are to challenge the status quo.

A further experience that I had some years ago whilst teaching at a prestigious south of England university relates to a discussion I was having with a group of qualified health professionals regarding the care of an unconscious individual suffering from hypoglycaemia, and clearly demonstrates the need for each of us to challenge the beliefs of our health or social care colleagues. The scene was a classroom of about 20 participants plus myself as the facilitator. As the discussion progressed on what actions and interventions should and should not be carried out, one participant stated out loud that they had been told that when you have such a situation, two chocolate bars should be inserted rectally!

At that point I had several thoughts and reactions. My immediate reaction was to look at the individual in such a way as to say 'You're having a laugh' (or words to that effect which I shall leave to your own imagination to work out). However, it became very obvious very quickly that the participant concerned was absolutely serious. My second reaction was to look at the rest of the participants who were having trouble stopping themselves falling off their chairs on to the floor in hysterics of laughter and I suppose, for them, it was one of those situations when you know you should not laugh but really wanted to. Then, and I have to be honest here in saying that my sense of humour took over and what came to mind was: what size of chocolate bars was this individual referring to? The other thing that came to mind was the sudden and horrific thought that this individual might one day be observed running down a supermarket isle shouting, 'Stand back!' with a chocolate bar or two in their hand(s) ready to administer them to an individual who appeared in need. It subsequently transpired that I had to explain in detail that under no circumstances should such an intervention ever be undertaken. What this experience shows quite clearly is that even those in health and social care can have some quite bizarre attitudes about what constitutes appropriate intervention.

It is unfortunate that when challenged, many health and social care professionals have a defensive reaction where they become hostile and sometimes abusive or make a complaint about your challenging them. In reality, they are the ones who should have the complaint made against them, not only for their unsafe behaviour, but also because of their unprofessional reaction to your challenge. Such negative reactions will serve to inhibit individuals form challenging further.

In the same vein, fear of being ostracised from a peer group can impact upon our willingness to challenge a colleague for similar reasons as being fearful of retribution from a higher authority. Humans, as a species, are social animals and have a deep-seated psychological need to feel part of a group. If we believe that an action we take will place our membership of a group under threat then it is likely that we will not take that action, but choose to selectively ignore it. However, in such a case we must always measure selectively ignoring another's unsafe behaviour against the issues of health and safety, human rights and our own standards of professionalism. If we selectively choose to ignore non-adherence to standard precautions are we being professional? Do we have the right to call ourselves a professional? In both cases the answer has to be 'No!'.

REFLECTION EXERCISE 12.10

Have you ever selectively ignored unsafe practice?

If your answer is yes then do you still have the right to consider yourself to be professional or refer to yourself as a professional?

Indifference and choosing to ignore what we observe can also be barriers to challenging the status quo. For example, although many health and social care professionals purport to care about patients and clients, I would suggest that in some cases their caring is borne out of social nicety and expectation. Now, at this point you may throw your arms up in horror at what I have just stated. However, in reflecting upon the idea of indifference, which may be defined as a *lack of interest* or *a lack of concern*, it can be linked to the ethics of what we do or do not do in the case of adhering to standard precautions. In reality many health and social care professionals care little for the ethics of what they do and perceive ethics as having no relevance (Seedhouse 1998); that is, constituting a necessary evil. Furthermore, based upon current levels of healthcare-acquired infection rates and non-adherence to standard precautions, one might surmise that health and social care professionals are, in fact, indifferent and care little for the patients and clients or – for that matter – each other's safety. As such, health and social care professionals may talk a lot about the importance of challenging the status quo, but in reality, where unsafe infection-control practice is concerned, they do not practice what they preach and as such indicate that they are indifferent about others' health and wellbeing. Indifference is therefore a barrier to challenging the status quo.

Finally, the attitude that 'It is not my responsibility' can serve to inhibit health and social care professionals challenging the status quo. For example, we are all told that as practitioners we are responsible for our actions and omissions – a point which is clearly identified within health and social care professional bodies' codes of conduct. This being the case, it allows health and social care professionals to generate dissonance-based (*see* Explanation box 12.1) and cognitively economic (*see* Explanation box 12.3) excuses as a means of justifying, not challenging, unsafe practice because they perceive it as not being their responsibility. However, as has been identified within much of this book, humans are extremely adept at generating what are, in essence, irrational and tunnel-visioned excuses to justify their actions and omissions. Furthermore, the attitude that 'It is not my responsibility' is, in itself, an example of dissonance-based and cognitively economic thinking. As a health or social care professional, if you observe a colleague failing to adopt standard precautions before interacting with a patient or client whilst knowing such an omission can cause harm, but do nothing about it, you are in error.

CONCLUSION

I hope I have raised your awareness of not only the importance of challenging the status quo, but also of the consequences of not doing so, and some of the reasons why such challenging does not occur.

REFERENCES

Adams B, Bromley B. *Psychology for Healthcare: key terms and concepts.* Basingstoke: Macmillan; 1998.

Department of Health. *The Health Act 2006: code of practice for the prevention and control of healthcare associated infections.* London: Department of Health; 2006.

Elliott P. Recognising the psychosocial issues involved in hand hygiene. *J R Soc Promo Health.* 2003; **123**(2): 88–94.

Elliott P. Understanding clinical supervision: a health psychology orientated process of person-centred development. In: Jasper M, editor. *Vital Notes for Nurses: professional development, reflection and decision-making.* Oxford: Blackwell Publishing; 2006.

Elliott P, BVS Training. *Effective Hand Hygiene* (DVD/training pack). London: BVS Training; 2005. Available at: www.bvs.co.uk/index.asp (accessed 25 Nov 2008).

Festinger L. Cognitive dissonance. *Sci Am.* 1962; **207**: 93–102.

Gardner H, Kornhaber ML, Wake WK. Intelligence: multiple perspectives. In: Atkinson RL, Atkinson RC, Smith E, *et al. Hilgard's Introduction to Psychology.* 13th ed. London: Harcourt College; 2000.

Graves N, Weinhold D, Tong E, *et al.* Effect of healthcare-acquired infection on length of hospital stay and cost. *Infect Cont Hosp Ep.* 2007; **28**(3): 280–92.

Grilli R, Lomas J. Evaluating the message: the relationship between compliance rate and the subject of a practice guideline. *Med Care.* 1994; **32**(3): 202–13.

Lawton R, Parker D. Procedures and the professional: the case of the British NHS. *Soc Sci Med.* 1999; **48**: 353–61.

Lawton R, Parker D. Judgments of the rule-related behaviour of healthcare professionals: an experimental study. *Br J Health Psych.* 2002; **7**(3): 253–65.

Neuberger J. Do we need a new word for patients?: let's do away with 'patients'. *BMJ.* 1999; **318**: 1756–8.

O'Dowd A. Nurses criticise poor hygiene practice among theatre staff. *Nurs Times.* 2006; **102**(16): 4.

Ogden J. *Health Psychology: a textbook.* 4th ed. Maidenhead: Open University Press/ McGraw-Hill; 2007.

Reason J, Parker D, Lawton R. Organisational controls and safety: the varieties of role-related behaviour. *J Occup Organ Psych.* 1998; **71**: 289–304.

Roth I, Frisby J. *Perception and Representation: a cognitive approach.* Milton Keynes: Open University; 1992.

Royal College of Nursing. *Wipe It Out: guidance on uniforms and clothing worn in the delivery of patient care.* London: Royal College of Nursing; 2007.

Seedhouse D. *Ethics: the heart of healthcare.* 2nd ed. Chichester: John Wiley and Sons; 1998.

Stone P, Clarke S, Cimiotti J, Correa-de-Araujo R. Nurses' working conditions: implications for infectious disease. *Emerg Infect Dis* (International Conference on Women and Infectious Diseases). 2004; **10**(11): 1984–9.

Storr J, Topley K, Privett S. The ward nurse's role in infection control. *Nurs Stand.* 2005; **19**(41): 56–64.

Taylor A. Global governance, international health law and WHO: looking towards the future. Geneva. *Bull World Health Organ.* 2002; **80**: 975–80.

Teale K. What's wrong with the wards? *BMJ.* 2007; **334**: 97.

Wallston K, Wallston B. Who is responsible for your health?: the construct of health locus of control. In: Sanders G, Suls J, editors. *Social Psychology of Health and Illness.* Hillsdale: Erlbaum; 1982.

Wilkinson R, Caulfield H. *The Human Rights Act: a practical guide for nurses.* Chichester: John Wiley; 2001.

CHAPTER 13

Raising public awareness: failure to inform, failure to protect and healthcare inequalities

Within this final chapter I intend to reflect upon the importance of public awareness and the public's right to know what they might expect from contact with health and social care professionals and healthcare providers. It is my intention to do this through providing topical examples where the health and wellbeing of patients and clients might have been affected as a result of failure to inform, failure to adequately protect and examples of healthcare inequalities. To this end, it is my intention not only to reflect upon issues within infection control, but also to take a broader perspective. In addition, I shall link these to the issues of human rights, health and safety and a number of the theories and approaches that I have identified throughout this book as being central to the psychosocial issues.

I will start by getting right to the heart of the matter. Currently, cross-infection rates, levels of non-adherence to standard precautions among health and social care workers, plus their dissonance-based (*see* Explanation box 13.1) irresponsible behaviour and the standards of cleanliness within many healthcare settings, constitute a considerable risk to the general population from contracting serious and life-threatening infections, which they did not have upon initial contact (Gould 2005).

EXPLANATION BOX 13.1 COGNITIVE DISSONANCE (FESTINGER 1962)

The concept of cognitive dissonance was originally identified by Festinger (1962), where he proposed that, at a psychological level, the individual will strive

---

to make consistent two or more things that would not naturally be so. In simple terms, dissonance effects are when an individual generates excuses to justify their previous behaviour or behaviour they wish or intend to carry out. Hand hygiene is a good example, where the individual understands its importance in reducing cross infection, yet fails to adequately follow the hand hygiene process. Thus the individual experiences conflict between knowing what they should do and what they actually do or want to do.

Such conflict would manifest as stress in the individual and in an attempt to reduce such stress the individual will generate an excuse or reason for failing to follow the hand hygiene process. Such an excuse may be blamed on time, work load or an irrational belief that meeting other's needs must take priority.

Serious and life-threatening infections can be described as *added extras* because many individuals who seek and receive health or social care interventions do not initially present with an infection. Yet as a consequence of interacting with health or social care workers, patients and clients experience added extras to the care and treatment they receive. Such added extras will, at best, have consequences for an individual's remaining life span. At worst, such added extras can be causal factors in the individual's death (Pittet and Donaldson 2005).

REFLECTION EXERCISE 13.1

Consider situations where an individual has sought health or social care intervention and, as a consequence of that, has contracted an added extra.

Reflect upon the ethics and morality of a situation where an individual seeks help and as a result is discharged with an added extra, or are forced, through no fault of their own, to spend a longer period of time receiving health or social care intervention than was initially necessary.

Can you think of any other organisations than those involved in the provision of health and social care who would impose such a negative added extra upon their consumers?

Individuals seek the interventions of health and social care workers and providers when they experience a health or social problem that they feel unable to resolve themselves. In doing this, they have the right to expect interventions that are professional, safe, ensure equity for all and do not breach their human or health and safety rights. Yet a look at the UK Healthcare Commission (2007), Health Protection Agency (2007) and the US Center for Disease

Control and Prevention (2007) websites clearly indicates that this is not always the case, with added extras such as MRSA, *C. difficile* and the norovirus constituting a serious problem (*CDR Weekly* 2005; Redelings, Sorvillo and Mascola 2007).

MRSA and *C. difficile* are perhaps the most well-known because of the amount of media coverage they have received. However, the norovirus can also present problems for public health and wellbeing because immunity is not long lasting. In addition, it is generally thought of as being a disease of winter and as such is not perceived as potentially serious because of the perception that winter is a season when people might expect to become ill. In contrast, MRSA and *C. difficile* are perceived to be with us all the time (which they are) as a result of the continuous media coverage they receive. Yet, as with the risks associated with MRSA and *C. difficile*, the general public should also be on their guard regarding the norovirus. For example, the primary route of transmission for the norovirus is fecal-oral (Koplan *et al.* 2001); therefore, health and social care professionals and patients/clients can spread this virus through a failure to adopt appropriate standard precautions.

The general public needs to be as assertive in ensuring that health and social care professionals adopt appropriate standard precautions as a preventative measure against the norovirus as they should be regarding MRSA and *C. difficile*. Health and social care organisations exist to provide a safe service to the general population – a service that individuals pay for either privately or through a variety of insurance payments. For example, within the UK, deductions are taken directly from salaries and wages under a National Insurance Scheme. Yet within the UK's National Health Service (NHS), those who pay for healthcare through this scheme are perceived by many as receiving their healthcare for free. This is not the case, but has resulted in inequalities related to the swiftness of healthcare intervention.

REFLECTION EXERCISE 13.2

Consider situations where, within your workplace, inequalities in health or social care could or do exist regarding those who pay by a National Insurance Scheme and those by private means.

Should a person's speed or quality of healthcare intervention be determined by the means by which they pay or how much they pay?

Let us consider two individuals with the same health problem. Individual 1 pays for their healthcare through the government-managed National Insurance

Scheme and as a consequence finds themselves in the position of having to wait weeks or even months to receive the treatment they need. In contrast, Individual 2 pays by private means and as such finds that they can be seen by the relevant health or social care professional within a much shorter period of time. The general population has a right to know that they are, for all intents and purposes, in a two-tier system – a system where how you pay and how much you pay, in many cases, determines the time span for interventions to occur. Clearly this is a system where some are more equal than others. However, in all fairness, the UK does at least guarantee all its citizens healthcare. In the US, the issue of health inequalities appears even greater as it is the only nation within the industrialised world that does not guarantee all its citizens healthcare (Thompson and Lee 2007). Such a guarantee is only afforded to the 'haves'; that is, those who can afford health insurance.

Skevington (1996) reflects upon the difference in interventions between men and women, for example, presenting with back or chest pain. Skevington identifies that men are sent for an electro-cardiogram (ECG), but when women present with such pain they are sent for laboratory tests. The implication is that chest pain in men is more genuine and objective, but in women is more subjective and hysteria-based, possibly as a result of them seeking healthcare intervention almost twice as much as men (Skevington 1996). In this way, women are clearly subject to inequalities in healthcare intervention because assumptions are being made about the nature and origins of a given health problem on the basis of gender. If the pain were the result of a cardiac problem, sending the individual for laboratory tests could be life-threatening because of the length of time involved in arranging such tests and the time it could take to receive the results. Although laboratory tests might ultimately reveal the presence of a cardiac problem, by the time this becomes apparent the individual could well have suffered serious harm.

In contrast, if the pain were the result of an infection and an ECG were performed, it would provide no indication that an infection was present. Again, the inequalities in healthcare would be the result of assumptions based upon gender stereotypes.

As an example, let us return to the idea of how we pay for our healthcare. Within this context, a stereotype held by a health or social care worker might centre around the cognitively economic belief (*see* Explanation box 13.2) that those who pay through National Insurance are of lower social status or economically poorer and are categorised as elderly or unemployed.

EXPLANATION BOX 13.2 COGNITIVE ECONOMY
(ROTH AND FRISBY 1992)

Cognitive economy is where an individual has become context-specific or tunnel-visioned in their perception of what is occurring around them and will fail to take into account the wider implications of their behaviour. For example, instead of being patient-centred, the individual will become task-orientated towards achieving a set of goals that will meet their own needs at the expense of everything else and the needs of others.

Example: In the case of standard precautions, the individual will be context-specific towards achieving their allocated work load and as a result of this may:
- fail to change their gloves between interventions;
- fail to undertake or to fully follow the hand hygiene process;
- fail to ensure that they have removed all the equipment they used following completion of a procedure.

In contrast, the same health or social care worker might also hold the cognitively economic belief that those who have private insurance are employed and earn a salary (paid monthly) as opposed to a wage (paid weekly); that they are of a higher social status; of greater intelligence; and are more articulate. However, as we have seen from previous chapters, none of these factors are good and reliable measures.

REFLECTION EXERCISE 13.3

Can you think of any situations where the gender of an individual could or has resulted in harm?

As a health or social care worker how does this make you feel?

As an individual of a particular gender how do you feel about such inequalities?

Have you ever judged another individual in a negative way as a result of their gender? (For example, 'man flu' or 'They're hormonal; it's that time of the month.')

Such assumptions are the result of health and social care workers drawing inferences based upon their prejudices and their attitudes towards a given individual, group or part of society. In providing an example here I would like to reflect upon a situation I observed many years ago in an accident and emergency department. It was late evening and nearing the end of a shift when an individual presented who was well-known to the department as living on the streets and being a regular at attending. The individual was complaining of cervical neck pain following a fall. However – and this is where all of us in health and social care have to be careful about letting our prejudices lead to inequalities of healthcare – the individual was told to sit in the waiting room. Eventually the individual was brought through and sat in a cubical to be seen by a doctor, but because this individual was well-known to the department, the general attitude was to perceive their need as of lesser importance.

Sometime later it was determined, rather nonchalantly, that perhaps they should be sent for an x-ray. The individual was given an x-ray request form and told to walk round to the x-ray department. A short time later, this individual wandered back into the cubical and handed over the x-ray film. As there had been no communication from the radiographer who took the x-ray, no particular urgency was afforded to looking at the film. When the film was eventually reviewed, it was discovered that the individual had a fracture of the third cervical vertebrae. At this point the motivation towards this individual increased ten-fold and in all my 37 years in nursing I have never seen a cervical collar applied to someone and them being immobilised on a trolley so quickly! Sadly, all those involved then focused primarily on covering their backs with dissonanced-based and cognitively economic excuses for their actions and omissions. Of course, what they should have done was had the professionalism to acknowledge their failings and adopt the attitude of 'What can we learn form this situation/experience?'.

On a personal note, I learnt two very valuable lessons from this experience, which have served me well throughout the whole of my career. First, pain and discomfort are what the patient or client says they are and not what we as health and social care professionals *think* they are. Second, never judge an individual by their appearance or the number of times they attend. Clearly the inequalities of healthcare that this individual experienced were the result of prejudicial and stereotypical attitudes held by those they encountered. In addition, there was a clear failure to protect the individual's health and well-being. Such prejudices and stereotyping arguably emanate from the processes of cognitive dissonance (*see* Explanation box 13.1), cognitive economy (*see* Explanation box 13.2) and unrealistic optimism (*see* Explanation box 13.3).

EXPLANATION BOX 13.3 UNREALISTIC OPTIMISM (OGDEN 2007)

Unrealistic optimism is where a health or social care professional becomes unrealistically optimistic regarding the risky situation they place themselves and others in as a result of behaviour that constitutes unsafe infection control practice in the form of failing to undertake standard precautions or through failing to follow the hand hygiene process.

Unrealistic optimism can be facilitated through lack of personal experience. For example, a health or social care professional who has no or little prior experience of a patient's or client's health being directly influenced by their failure to adopt appropriate standard precautions will likely believe two things (Elliott 2003):

1 There is no risk, or the risk of cross infecting others is so insignificant that it simply does not matter.
2 Even if there is a risk it will not happen to them. That is, even if the individual involved in healthcare does cross infect others they will rationalise that is was not their fault (*see* Explanation box 13.1) or they will not be found out and held responsible and therefore, who cares?

Such prejudicial and stereotypical attitudes may also be perceived as breaches of the individual's human rights; for example, an individual's right to life (Wilkinson and Caulfield 2001), where the failure to act appropriately regarding what the individual communicated could have impacted upon their survival.

REFLECTION EXERCISE 13.4

As a health or social care worker, have you ever judged an individual in such a way that it could have or did result in them experiencing physical or psychological harm?

For example, have you ever made assumptions about the genuineness of what an individual was telling you?

There is little doubt that the care many patients and clients receive is significantly below an acceptable standard, irrespective of whether they are paying consumers or not. I can think of no other organisation than those providing health and social care where, in terms of infection prevention, the level of consumer care provided constitutes such a consistent and unresolved threat to the general population's health and safety.

This reflection exercise is in two parts.

At this point, take some time to reflect upon the above paragraph.

Part 1:

From your perspective as a health or social care worker, how do you feel about the public's right to know about the risks they are at from contracting an added extra, which may have a permanent impact upon their future life span or even their life?

Should the public be made aware or should the information be kept from them?

Write down your feelings. Having done that, go and do something else for an hour, then come back (*but do not look at your notes from undertaking Part 1*).

Part 2:

From your perspective as a member of the general population, do you feel you have the right to be told about the risks you are at from contracting an infection when seeking or receiving health or social care intervention?

Or would you rather not be told and as such be unable to protect yourself from harm?

Write down your feelings.

Now compare your notes from Part 1 and Part 2 and see if there are similarities/differences.

Where such consistently poor consumer care is concerned, the importance of providing the general population with appropriate information is paramount. This is particularly so when considered within the context of individuals needing to make choices that may directly impact upon their self-preservation and right to life (Wilkinson and Caulfield 2001).

In order to make choices, general populations not only need to be informed of situations or events where health and social care workers and healthcare providers have failed to maintain appropriate standards of infection prevention, but also such information should be made available promptly. Failing to provide information can be harmful (Williamson 2005). Threats to public health can result not only from failures to maintain appropriate standards but also from a failure to inform within a reasonable time (measuring days and not weeks, months or years).

Furthermore, where an organisation at a collective level fails to inform its consumers or does very little towards responding to significant problems that could or have resulted in harm to members of the population, then that may be deemed to be organisational silence (Henriksen and Dayton 2006).

There is, of course, the issue of public confidence. For example, any health or social care provider who withholds information that prevents or restricts members of the population from taking reasonable steps to protect their health and wellbeing will inevitably leave themselves open to significant media interest when found out. In addition, such a provider will lose public trust and credibility.

However, what must be remembered is that when a health or social care provider's failings are brought into the public domain – particularly where serious harm or injury has occurred – it is likely that they will be castigated. Although such castigation may well be justified, it must be tempered against the time lapse between when the failings occurred and when they became public. In some cases, during such a time lapse many changes and improvements may have been implemented by the organisation in question, and those bringing the information into the public arena and those reporting it must therefore take this into consideration to ensure a fair and unbiased perspective is given. This will allow the general public to make an informed judgement.

Failure on the part of an individual health or social care professional, a healthcare provider or other relevant organisation to promptly inform the public could have implications regarding an individual's human right to receive relevant information (Wilkinson and Caulfield 2001); that is, the right to receive information without interference by public authority.

Interference by a public authority might be perceived as withholding information or taking an excessive amount of time to make such information available to the general public. For whatever reason, a failure to promptly inform the public of events that could have a significant impact upon the public's health and wellbeing clearly has ethical implications and would not constitute acting in a person-centred way.

REFLECTION EXERCISE 13.6

Have you ever withheld information from a patient or client regarding a potential or actual cross-infection risk?

For example, have you ever failed to adopt appropriate standard precautions when you have known you should have done so?

If so how did you justify your decision?

Did part of your justification include admitting to the patient or client that you had not adopted standard precautions properly?

In reflecting do you feel that the patient or client had a right to know about your failure?

How ethical was your decision?

Having completed this exercise, I strongly recommend that you read the Gallagher and Levinson (2005) paper.

A general principle of health and safety centres on the responsibility of both individuals and organisations to protect others. However, if the public are not informed until sometime after an event then that would seem to raise questions related to helping the public to adequately protect themselves.

The public's right to know and be provided with appropriate information goes beyond clinical health and social care settings; for example, within higher education settings where the education and skills training of future health and social care professionals occurs. Lecturing staff, like their clinical and social care counterparts, do on occasions attend work and come into close contact with others knowing full well that they are unwell and potentially infectious. Yet in doing so, one can only assume that they care little for the health and wellbeing of those they will be likely to cross infect. Again, in justifying their actions it is likely they will establish dissonance-based excuses (*see* Explanation box 13.1), which they will further support with unrealistically optimistic beliefs (*see* Explanation box 13.3).

Some examples are:

'When I am teaching and know I am unwell, I keep my distance from the students. Therefore the risk of cross infecting them is negligible.' In the case of this dissonance-based excuse the individual is unrealistically optimistic regarding the potential for airborne transmission – something that is frequently forgotten when individuals sneeze or cough.

'I know I am unwell and infectious, but if I do not go to work I will be letting my patients and colleagues down.' In the case of this dissonance-based excuse, the individual is unrealistically optimistic about letting people down. Yet by going to work in an infectious state they are letting their patients, clients, colleagues and students down because of the cross-infection risk they will constitute.

The generation of such dissonance-based excuses serves to allow the health or social worker to place their own needs before the needs of others and yet they will energetically argue the importance of being person-centred in their professional activities. The placing of such needs above the needs of others is currently an endemic practice among health and social care workers.

REFLECTION EXERCISE 13.7

If you are a health or social care professional, either within a clinical or education arena, how do you feel about others coming to work and potentially cross infecting you?

In the past, if you have been guilty of such behaviour, what do you think you are teaching your students about the ethics of cross infecting others?

Do you think the general public has a right to know about your questionable behaviour?

The public's right to know can also be seen as an issue of person-centred care. The essence of this is that health and social care workers, their employers and government bodies, have a moral, ethical and professional duty to protect the public from physical, psychological and social harm.

The principle of being person-centred is about informing without frightening. Yet when there is an extensive period of time between an adverse situation being discovered and it being placed within the public domain this does not constitute person-centred practice.

CONCLUSION

In this chapter I have reflected upon how the health, safety and welfare of the general public and their human rights can be adversely affected through the withholding of information, the time span taken to place information in the public domain and through the instigation of health inequalities. In whatever capacity we are involved in health and social care, we must always be on our guard against such influences.

REFERENCES

Centers for Disease Control and Prevention. 2007. Available at: www.cdc.gov/Diseases Conditions/ (accessed 25 Nov 2008).

CDR Weekly 2005. Results of the first year of mandatory Clostridium difficile reporting: January to December 2004. Commun Dis Rep CDR Wkly. 25 Aug; 15(34).

Elliott P. Recognising the psychosocial issues involved in hand hygiene. J R Soc Promo Health. 2003; 123(2): 88–94.

Festinger L. Cognitive dissonance. Sci Am. 1962; 207: 93–102.

Gallagher T, Levinson W. Disclosing harmful medical errors to patients: a time for professional action. Arch Intern Med. 2005; 165(16): 1819–24.

Gould D. Infection control: the environment and service organisation. Nurs Stand. 2005; 20(5): 57–65.

Healthcare Commission. 2007. Available at: http://2007ratings.healthcarecommission.org.uk/homepage.cfm (accessed 25 Nov 2008).

Health Protection Agency. 2007. Available at: www.hpa.org.uk/ (accessed 25 Nov 2008).

Henriksen K, Dayton E. Organizational silence and hidden threats to patient safety. *Health Serv Res.* 2006; **41**(4 Part 2): 1539–54.

Kaplan J, Hughes J, LeDuc J, *et al.* Norwalk-like viruses: public health consequences and outbreak management. *CDC, U.S. Department of Health and Human Services.* 2001; 50(RR-9).

Ogden J. *Health Psychology: a textbook.* 4th ed. Maidenhead: Open University Press/McGraw-Hill; 2007.

Pittet D, Donaldson L. Clean care is safer care: the first global challenge of the WHO world alliance for patient safety. *Infect Cont Hosp Ep.* 2005; **26**(11): 891–4.

Redelings M, Sorvillo F, Mascola L. *Increase in* Clostridium difficile-*related mortality rates, United States, 1999–2004.* 2007. Available at: www.cdc.gov/eid/content/13/9/1417.htm (accessed 25 Nov 2008).

Roth I, Frisby J. *Perception and Representation: a cognitive approach.* Milton Keynes: Open University; 1992.

Skevington S. *Psychology of Pain.* Chichester: John Wiley; 1996.

Thompson J, Lee V. The effect of health insurance disparities on the healthcare system. *AORN.* 2007; **85**(5): 745–56.

Wilkinson R, Caulfield H. *The Human Rights Act: a practical guide for nurses.* Chichester: John Wiley; 2001.

Williamson C. Withholding policies from patients restricts their autonomy. *BMJ.* 2005; **331**(7524): 1078–80.

Book summary

I hope this book has helped you to realise that infection control (or infection prevention as it now starting to be called) is far more complex than you might have originally imagined.

The importance of adopting a biopsychosocial approach in the way you perceive and practise infection control/prevention is paramount to the health, wellbeing and survival of those you interact with.

Developing your skills of self-awareness is vital in reducing the risk of complacency setting in regarding how you carry out or adopt infection control/prevention measures, such as standard precautions. Humans are habitual, dissonanced-based, cognitively economic and unrealistically optimistic in nature, and as such are extremely prone to complacency in what they do. Do not be fooled into believing that because you have done something many times before, the next time you do the same thing it will be carried out in a safe manner. Reflection both in and on action are vital elements in ensuring that you maintain safe levels of practice. **Think, 'What have I just done and what am I about to do? What infection prevention measures do I need to implement?'**

Standard precautions are there to be applied all the time and not simply when you happen to remember or can be bothered! Adopting standard precautions is not just about protecting others from the risks of cross infection; it is also about self-preservation! Remember, lack of time is never a valid or reliable excuse for failing to adopt standard precautions.

React positively when you observe dangerous practice in others. Intervene and challenge the individual(s) concerned. Do not ignore it, walk away or suddenly develop selective blindness. It is about having the professionalism and moral fibre to stand up and be counted.

In brief:
➤ Think about reducing infection.
➤ Reflect upon your own infection control/prevention practices.

➤ Think about the importance of reducing cross infection through such measures as standard precautions.
➤ React positively when you observe others adopting dangerous practices that could harm others, infringe their human rights, contravene health and safety regulations or your employer's prescriptive rules.

Infection control and its prevention are everyone's problem and everyone's responsibility. Which side of the fence will you sit on: the selectively blind or the interventionists'?

It is my hope that you found reading this book not only a challenging experience, but also an enlightening one. As I indicated at the beginning of the book, I deliberately set out to challenge your attitudes and beliefs, the status quo in general and to push the frontiers of thinking where infection control is concerned and for doing this I make no apology. Currently, where infection control is concerned, those in health and social care are actively contributing to the demise of others.

Finally, having read this book, I hope that your approach to infection control has taken a significant leap forward and that your practice – no matter how good or bad it may have been in the past – will reflect such a leap.

Where infection control is concerned, are you made of the right stuff?
Do you have what it takes to make a sustained difference?

Index

Entries in **bold** denote text in figures, boxes or lists.